Personal RESILIENCE

Also by Peter Tarlow

Personal Reconstruction

Twenty Years of Tourism Tidbits: The Book

The Twenty-Twenty Election: A Survivor's Guide

and many other books about security of tourism and sports

Also by Séverine Obertelli

Mindful Time Management

To Bernard,
a loving neighbour
Severine

Personal
RESILIENCE

FIRST EDITION

SURVIVAL STRATEGIES FOR PANDEMIC TIMES

Peter Tarlow
&
Séverine Obertelli

Quest Publishing • Miami, Florida

Inquiries should be directed to:

Quest Publishing
2655 S. Le Jeune Road, Suite 500
Coral Gables, FL 33134 U.S.A.
Tel. +1 305.779.3069 • Fax +1 305.901.2120
email: editor@quest-publishing.com

Print ISBN: 978-0-9769416-4-4
ePub ISBN: 978-0-9769416-5-1
Library of Congress Control Number 2021906369

Editor: Jacques Island

First Edition: April 2021

10 9 8 7 6 5 4 3 2 1

Visit us on the web at quest-publishing.com.

We dedicate this book
to all who have perished
during the Covid-19 pandemic
of 2020 and 2021.

Contents

Questions

25 QUESTIONS ABOUT HEALTH IN A PANDEMIC

25 QUESTIONS TO EXPLORE SPIRITUALITY

25 QUESTIONS FOR SOCIAL SURVIVAL IN A PANDEMIC

25 QUESTIONS ABOUT MONEY ISSUES IN A PANDEMIC

Foreword

Humanity suffers from crises and disasters constantly. The breadth of the latest health crisis—the COVID-19 pandemic—has affected all corners of the world and has caused millions of deaths, and so many more victims who have survived its worst effects.

Nonetheless, the survivors still suffer long-lasting physical or mental health issues from it. Those "lucky" enough to have suffered only mild cases, or managed to avoid infection altogether, are still victims because of the social and economic distresses that the pandemic has caused. Even so, it's becoming more apparent each passing day of the pandemic that people who contract only a mild or asymptomatic case of this disease may not be out of the woods after the initial bout. Some may still suffer lingering, unexpected, long-lasting harm to their health as the virus progresses through its hosts.

This book leads to a better understanding of the effects that pandemics have on us by exploring four areas of our human condition—health, spirituality, social issues, and finances—and offers strategies through 100 questions and answers about living through a pandemic.

It is the cooperative work of two noted authors and motivational speakers who focus on personal and organizational resilience: Dr. Peter Tarlow, a world-renowned speaker and a columnist about philosophy, religion, and risk management; and

Séverine Obertelli, an accomplished business entrepreneur focused on the development of leadership skills and strategies for individuals and businesses.

Their insights will lift your spirits as you face the ongoing pandemic or any other health crisis that's sure to happen again; and they'll equip you to better handle the hardships of prolonged confinements, restricted socialization—or a medical battle, should an invisible, microbial enemy invade your body.

Personal Resilience is a standalone work specifically focused on pandemics. It is meant to be read by itself. But it can also serve as a supplement to either of two other books in our growing risk and crisis management series: the seminal books of *Personal Reconstruction* and *Your Plan is Your Parachute*, both of which only touch on pandemics as one of the many crises that can affect us.

By the end of *Personal Resilience*, you'll have a better understanding of a pandemic's effects on our minds and our health, and you'll have simple, useful strategies to manage the stresses of these far-reaching health crises.

Jacques Island
Chief Editor

Prologue

PERSONAL CRISES IN THE TIMES OF COVID-19

When my colleagues and I first considered writing this book or its earlier companion *Personal Reconstruction*, no one had ever heard of coronavirus or COVID-19. Just a mere three years ago it was unimaginable that we'd be confined to our homes "sheltered-in-place," and toilet paper would become almost more valuable than petroleum.

At the start of last year very few foresaw that in just a few short weeks boom economies would be on the verge of collapse, that international borders would be reestablished and globalization might well come to its end. But in mere weeks, by February of 2020, our lives had changed.

Around the world, constitutional and democratic liberties gave way to the effects of a worldwide pandemic. In this new world, churches and synagogues switched to online worship, parks and restaurants closed, sporting events ceased to exist and in some places traditional voting gave way to health concerns.

The pandemic also produced new heroes. People who worked in the medical profession became international superstars, and the public gained a great deal of respect and admiration for those manning the front lines: from truck drivers to postal workers, from cashiers to law enforcement officers and firefighters.

For many who were familiar with the work of the Nobel Prize winner for literature, author Gabriel García Márquez, it felt like we had entered into the pages of his world famous book, *El Amor En Los Tiempos Del Cólera.* Although lost in English translation, Spanish speakers immediately caught the title's irony. By his book's title, did García Márquez' mean *Love In the Times of Cholera* or *Love In the Times of Rage*? Or was it *Love In the Season of Illness*? Or, did he mean them all? This multiple play-on-words and the irony expressed in Garcia Marquez' book seems to be a perfect fit for our times as the world is raged by today's "cholera," the sofocating *coronavirus*.

Despite the fact that in 2018 none of us had any idea of the obstacles we would face just two years later the basic premises of this book are as relevant and meaningful as ever. We designed *Personal Reconstruction* and this book, *Personal Resilience*, under the premise that there are four major pillars that cause personal crises: those provoked by economic, legal, psychological, and spiritual problems. In reality often these problems interconnect, and the 2019 pandemic that has stretched into 2021 has been triggering crises in all four pillars on innumerable people everywhere.

For four decades as a rabbi in a congregational setting, a university setting, and as a volunteer police chaplain, I saw how these issues caused problems and how people often felt so overwhelmed by them that they felt helpless in reconstructing their lives.

The coronavirus pandemic has exacerbated the personal crises of the young whose busy social lives have been truncated, and it has been particularly cruel to those in crowded living and working facilities, and to the individuals confined to detention centers.

The reason that my colleagues and I wrote this book was to help people recognize the sources of their problems before they became too big to handle. When handled quickly problems don't manifest themselves in negative behaviors or consequences. Another purpose was to show how not to lose hope but rather learn from mistakes and avoid repeating them again.

Today our world faces greater challenges then ever before. We do not know if COVID-19 will become a recurring part of our lives or if it will pass on into history. What we do know is that in the words of the Rabbi Tarfon (Second Century), "It is not your responsibility to finish the work of perfecting the world, but you are not free to desist from it either" (Pirke Avot 2:21).

Rabbi Peter Tarlow
College Station, Texas
March 2021

CHAPTER

1

INTRODUCTION

Humpty Dumpty sat on a wall,
Humpty Dumpty had a great fall;
All the king's horses and all the king's men
Couldn't put Humpty together again.

—Mother Goose
Nursery Rhyme

IN 2018, THREE of my colleagues and I published a book entitled *Personal Reconstruction*. We wrote the book only a few years ago, but now more than a year into the COVID-19 pandemic, it feels as if we had written that book during another age. We wrote it long before anyone had heard of COVID-19 or contemplated how it would change the world and each of our lives.

Now we are well into an age of pandemics, and more than personal reconstruction is needed. In this new era we need a sense of *resiliency*, an ability as the old Timex watch commercial used to say, "to keep on ticking" no matter what the world throws at us. As the American patriot Thomas Pain wrote in December of 1776 as the nation faced the onslaught of British forces, "These are the times that try men's souls."

Today we once again are forced to fight a foreign foe. Instead of British soldiers attempting to devastate the land, we must face an invisible enemy.

Today's enemy is one that is much more powerful and deadly than the British occupation forces of the late 18th and early 19th centuries. This invisible enemy attacks not merely our bodies and our economy but also our souls. It has forced us to ask new and deeper questions about our place in the world, our legal system, our economy and how we deal with others and ourselves psychologically.

THE GENESIS OF A PANDEMIC

When the world first grappled with COVID-19, then called coronavirus, no one understood its impact or the science behind it. Although the "2020 pandemic" was not the first one to impact the world, in almost every conceivable way not only were we in the United States woefully unprepared, but the same can also be said for most of the world.

We were cognizant of the tragic deaths caused by the 1918 Spanish flu, but perhaps our arrogance, based on the belief that science held the answer to all maladies, blinded us to the possibility that another major pandemic might occur.

We were aware that even in the later part of the 20th century and first decades of the 21st century the world had experienced epidemics, but these epidemics tended to be confined to a particular area, were somewhat short-lived, and on a global scale did minimal economic damage. Many political leaders had come to believe, or had convinced themselves, that a worldwide pandemic was a thing of the past.

In fact, the average person living in the developed world viewed such epidemics as H1N1, Ebola, or SARS as diseases happening in underdeveloped regions to be read about in a newspaper or as news to be viewed on television. Until the advent of COVID-19 most people assumed that these were diseases that occurred in far-off places and would most likely never impact their lives.

Before continuing, it would be wise to take a quick detour and provide a few words about the terms epidemic and pandemic. Currently epidemiologists use four words to classify or describe the outbreak of major diseases: epidemic, pandemic, endemic and outbreak. Intermountain Healthcare describes the difference between these four words:

- "AN EPIDEMIC is a disease that effects a large number of people within a community, population or region.

- "A PANDEMIC is an epidemic that's spread over multiple countries or continents.

- "ENDEMIC is something that belongs to a particular people or country.

- "AN OUTBREAK is a greater-than-anticipated increase in the number of endemic cases. It can also be a single case in a new area. If it's not quickly controlled, an outbreak can become an epidemic."

Using these definitions we can state that COVID-19 is the first major pandemic that the world has known since the 1918 Spanish flu, a worldwide disease that occurred over a century ago. It is estimated that the so-called Spanish influenza might have killed as many as fifty million people ("Spanish Flu"). It also had little to do with Spain!

Although COVID-19 has killed a smaller percentage of the world's population than did other past pandemics, its economic impact has been both devastating and universal. This fact is especially important in light of the fact that we now live in a globalized and highly interconnected world. For the first time in history, the world's economy basically shut down due to an illness rather than due to a war. In 2020 we saw more people thrown out of work than at any other time since the Great Depression of the 1930s.

HOW THIS PANDEMIC IS CHANGING SOCIETY

The still unknown aspects of COVID-19 have changed almost every aspect of our lives from the way we socialize to the way some of us can work, from our belief in science to the way that we gain spiritual health, from our trust in government to our understanding of self-reliance. For example, on the economic side, COVID-19 split the world between those who could "work from home" or at a social distance and those who could not and now found their income at least temporarily cancelled.

Small business people, store owners, and many medical personnel found themselves in a different reality from government bureaucrats and academics. The former became the new unemployed while the latter was encouraged to work from home and in many ways also saw the shut down as a reprieve from commuting. Small business people, hoteliers, restaurateurs, and people who provide travel services suddenly found their businesses closed and they suffered from economic hardships and psychological anxiety.

These forced shutdowns resulted in a new class system, which we might differentiate by those who could—and those who could not—telecommute.

This new class system might or might not be temporary and we do not yet know the full extent of its psychological, political and social consequences. We do not know either the impact of distance learning on children and if the closure of schools might reinforce or create new forms of classism.

Moreover, not all who could not telecommute necessarily suffered. Many major actors and sports figures are so wealthy that they could easily ride out the economic storm. On the other hand, many struggling actors and others in these industries' support groups such as stagehands and cleaning personnel lost both their paychecks and dignity.

Many people in the Western world, and not just in the United States, are facing the new reality that their nations are divided into a new set of social and economic groupings. At the time of this book's writing no one knows these new groupings' consequences on society and its political structure. We might borrow the terminology of these new groupings from the "Ancien Régime" of pre-revolutionary France. Then society was divided into three "estates." Then the first estate was composed of the clergy, the second was composed of the nobility and the third estate was composed of the commoners.

Today the first estate consists of people working for governments, multinational large corporations, academia, large retail and on-line shopping centers, and the wealthy retired. The shelter-in-place orders minimally impacted these people.

The second estate is now composed of workers whom the state determined were not essential. Those falling into the second estate are small business owners, many service providers, people working in restaurants, hotels and transportation and the poor retired. The shelter-in-place orders meant that these people were not only negatively economically impacted by the orders but also psychologically impacted as no one knows the full extent of the damage of being classified as "non-essential."

As in Medieval France, the third estate consists of everyone else. This estate includes the very poor, the homeless, baby sitters and home cleaning services, and perhaps agricultural workers. Some in this third "estate" continued to work, others ceased working and some find themselves living on the margins of society. COVID-19 did not impact everyone in the third estate. For example, some of the homeless were moved into upscale hotels and replaced those who had paid hundreds of dollars a night.

No matter into which estate a person fell, the shelter-in-place and fear of illnesses impacted almost everyone. Children missed school and parents became stay-at-home teachers, camp-counselors, and social directors. Food shopping became an adventure and curbside service became the new normal.

This new reality fell especially hard on younger children and their parents, older adults and those with prior health conditions. All these people suddenly found themselves confined to their homes.

Home confinement saved many from the threat of COVID-19 but in many cases these same protected people now suffered from extreme loneliness. Others, who lived in senior citizen centers were cut off from families and until this day no one knows how many might have died in these senior citizen locations due to policy decisions made by several governors.

In the following chart we breakdown the U.S. population by age cohorts and list each group's major COVID-19 challenge. It is worth noting that many of the challenges impact more than one cohort.

AGE COHORT	MAJOR COVID-19 PROBLEM/CHALLENGE
Very young children	Boredom, lack of friends, parents' frustration
Middle age children (Junior High)	Education by electronics, lack of socialization, lack of sports, frustration with parents
Teenage children	Loss of a year of schooling, social isolation, developmental impairment
Adults	Face both family and economic problems. Had to learn to divide time between child caring functions for many new economic realities. At the same time had the burden of absentee caring for elderly parents fall on their shoulders
Senior citizens	Issue of loneliness, lack of mobility and cabin fever, and inability to get non-COVID-19 medical attention

The above table is one among the many that might demonstrate how the pandemic impacted different cross-sections of the nation's population. As of the writing of this book, it is still too soon to determine if COVID-19 was an anomaly and that the world will soon return to what it called "normal" or a tipping point that changed the economic, political, and social structure forever—what is now being called "the new normal." We do not know if COVID-19 represents a new period in public health, a time when the world will need to face multiple and ongoing pandemics or if we shall be able to overcome the challenge and put "Humpty Dumpty" back together again.

This book then is more than a mere survival tool. It is a guide to re-enforce the most important tool that human beings have: their ability to be resilient, to adapt to new realities and to create hope where there was once despair.

The book's goal is to provide readers the ability to transform negative moments into positive outcomes. Its goal is help each person to refuse to allow the current situation to defeat him or her, but rather to find the inner strength as the old saying goes: to take lemons and turn them into lemonade or as the 19th century French poet and thinker Victor Hugo said: "Even the darkest night will end and the sun will rise." COVID-19 will end and the sun shall surely shine again.

OUTLINE OF THIS BOOK

So now we begin the searching knowing that these questions are not the end of the journey but its beginning and each of us is on a collective yet personal journey as we seek personal resilience in a time of pandemics and crises.

We have not written this book in a way that each chapter must be read in chronological order. Instead, the reader is invited to wade into it as he or she chooses. We have organized the book as a series of questions and answers, and we then grouped these questions and answers by themes.

This book will not cover every COVID-19 theme but instead is meant to present broad outlines and methodologies that will permit the reader to think for him or herself, debate with the book and find his or her own answers.

We want to caution the reader that this book does not present specific financial or medical advice. We cannot emphasize enough that before acting the reader should consult a trained legal, medical, finance or psychological professional. The material presented here is a commonsense approach but in no way should substitute for professional advice. The information contained in this book then is solely meant to activate deep questions but not to provide specific answers.

For specific questions of spirituality it is also advised to consult with the individual's clergy or religious specialist. It should be noted that different traditions often hold different answers to similar situations and in no way does this book purport to provide the correct answer in all circumstances.

Lastly, this book is written from an American perspective. This does not mean that it is not valid for people who live outside of the borders of the United States. It does explain why the examples given are American examples and the spelling and grammar reflect American usage.

CHAPTER

2

STAYING HEALTHY

THE INSPIRATIONAL SPEAKER and author Renée Trudeau writes that "Nurturing yourself is not selfish—it's essential to your survival and your well–being" (Uliano). The maintaining of health and wellness during a pandemic must be our first priority. Without our health, the other aspects of living through a pandemic become meaningless.

Surviving a pandemic means first staying healthy. Airlines teach us this basic rule when in their pre-liftoff briefings; they remind us that if oxygen is needed we need to put our masks on first and only then to aid those around us. The airline's logic is simple, aid providers can only be useful if they take care of themselves. Without that basic principle, the help provider is useless to everyone else.

During a pandemic our lives are not that different from being on an airplane. Let's consider a typical family with young children. In our hypothetical typical family, the parents are to the family what the pilots are to an airplane. Just as in the case of an airplane's pilots, if the parents are not well then they cannot take care of others in the household. In order to keep the household functioning, the family's "captains" must first be well.

HEALTHY BEHAVIOR DURING A PANDEMIC

Staying well during a pandemic is a challenge. Not only do we have our normal responsibilities but all sorts of new challenges also arise. These challenges are physical and psychological, spiritual and economic. For example, when children cannot go to school parents take on multiple added responsibilities. They must become full-time teachers and "camp directors," they might have additional cleaning, and might have to deal with economic challenges for which they were unprepared. Parents soon become tired and at times their fatigue overwhelms them both physically and emotionally. Even a simple shopping excursion becomes a challenge especially for parents of young children.

In our highly spread-out society parents might not have anyone with whom to leave children. Yet, to keep their children safe they must avoid becoming infected when they venture out to public places to shop for groceries, or run other necessary errands, or work. To add to the difficulties, many single parents run households, and this fact alone means that the single mother or father may never be off duty.

These additional chores and responsibilities can often mean that many people become so exhausted that basic health considerations are forgotten or overlooked. The result is not only that caregivers become sick and the entire households falter, but also those living alone become dependent on the goodwill of friends and neighbors.

Hygiene

During a pandemic it becomes more important than ever to take responsibility for our health and set examples for others. It is not an easy task to maintain a sense of health and dignity when we are scared, exhausted and see no light at the end of a tunnel. Yet we have no choice; during a pandemic it is more necessary than ever that we not only practice proper health habits, like good personal hygiene, but also make sure that each of us becomes an example for others. Good examples come less from what we say and more from what we do.

It is for this reason that perhaps the number one health threat during a pandemic is losing a sense of self. Because we are under pressure we often forget that all of us need to eat well, exercise, get sunshine and fresh air, and sleep. Doing all this is not easy, but it is essential. These actions might not prevent you from falling ill, but not doing them will increase your chances of becoming ill.

> "... perhaps the number one health threat during a pandemic is losing a sense of self."

The COVID-19 pandemic taught many of us the importance of learning to be less of a perfectionist and more flexible. Being at home meant that we had to learn to be more efficient, better time managers and then, after working for eight to ten hours, to stop and relax.

Sleep

From a health perspective sleep is more essential than ever during these stressful coronavirus times. Sleep allows the body to refresh itself, to heal the "wounds" of yesterday and to garner the strength necessary for the next day. For this reason, and especially during a pandemic, at least seven hours of sleep are essential for everyone. If sleeping seven or eight hours through the night becomes impossible then try to nap for an hour or two during the afternoon.

Anyone who has ever lived in Latin America can testify to the value of the siesta. Not only do siestas add to our relaxation and sleep quotient, but they also lower stress and put things back into perspective. The less stress we have the better we will perform and the more resilient our bodies can be to fight off disease.

Isolation

Pandemics and social isolation reinforce the maxim that human beings are social animals and few if any of us are designed to live in isolation. In times of a pandemic it is essential to accept the fact that no one person can do everything. We all need others to get through our increasingly difficult daily tasks.

During a pandemic there is not only the issue of additional household chores but there is also the fact that many of our support systems simply cease to exist. Things break or go wrong. In less trying times we call for a plumber or electrician as a matter of course. Not so in times of pandemics when our support systems begin to crumble and finding people from those who mow yards to people who fix things that break become challenges. We begin to question if we should allow these people into our homes or if we have to become jacks-of-all trades?

Even if we have the knowledge to fix or repair household equipment, care for the yard, and clean the house, how do we find the time to accomplish these additional tasks? Moreover, there are still personal needs that need to be attended to: during a pandemic we get sick or suffer an accident, need a haircut, require a dental appointment, and desperately need social interaction. And all these things can be big challenges during a pandemic.

THE CHANGING INFORMATION LANDSCAPE

We live in a world dominated by the desire for precise short answers and instant solutions. Unfortunately, when facing a new pandemic neither is possible. Although modern medicine has produced many miracles, the fact is that there is much information that medical experts do not know. For example, during the COVID-19 pandemic medical experts shared with the public their best advice based on the data that they had at that moment. As the situation changed, or as we learned more about the virus, medical experts changed or updated their advice.

These updates were not an attempt by medical experts to mislead the public. They were simply giving their best advice with the information that they had at the time. This need to give information as it is learned puts medical experts in a moral and political bind: not to share their best information is simply wrong, but today's correct information might not be tomorrow's best information and these changes lead to public frustration or even anger.

A perfect example of the public's frustration during the COVID-19 pandemic was the issue of face masks. During the early stages of the pandemic the medical profession gave conflicting advice regarding the use or non-use of face masks. This was merely the result of the fact that the medical profession's information was fluid and hospital personnel desperately needed these face masks. As medical experts discovered new information and the hospital situation stabilized the experts changed their advice.

> "[Changing science] updates [are] not an attempt by medical experts to mislead the public. They [are] simply giving their best advice with the information that they [have] at the time."

We tend to forget that medicine is not pure science but rather it is a combination of art plus science. Doctors learn through trial and error, but humans are not machines and there is more to healing than mere formulas.

In the case of a new pandemic doctors are often learning from each other as they attempt to treat patients. For example, in March of 2020 doctors at John Hopkins University's medical research center reached out to colleagues from around the world. Sharon Begley reported in STAT Magazine that

"When facing a global crisis, sharing of medical and scientific information is invaluable if we are to save lives and halt the pandemic as quickly as possible."

The issue of conflicting medical advice is not new. What perhaps is new is the public's understandable lack of patience and fears.

For decades insurance companies have suggested that patients get a second opinion. What this request means is that, in a world of new medical issues, the public should balance what is the current medical advice with what each individual, upon study and careful reflection, believes to be the correct option.

FEARING MEDICAL INSUFFICIENCIES

To a great extent pandemics create medical fear. That is to say that as doctors spend more of their time on the pandemic and access to medical treatment becomes increasingly limited we not only fear the pandemic but other medical issues. During pandemics medical personnel must create forms of triage: the need to give priorities to medical cases according to the case's severity. Often to preserve hospital beds elective surgeries are put on hold, doctors by necessity see fewer patients and medicine moves from the professional to the untrained.

This need for self-medical sufficiency often leaves many of us feeling adrift. Pharmacists become "doctors" and we fall back on folk medicine. The

Centers for Disease Control and Prevention (CDC) in Atlanta recognized this problem when it stated that "A consequence of the pandemic has been the under-utilization of important medical services for patients with non-COVID-19-related urgent and emergent health needs (CDC "Food," "Framework," "How to"). As the pandemic continues, healthcare systems must balance the need to provide necessary services while minimizing risk to patients and healthcare personnel."

Unfortunately the number one healthcare provider during pandemics for lack of other options might have to be an untrained family member or a friend. Because there might be a lack of access to medical professionals that are dealing with the pandemic's life-threatening illness, other illnesses or injuries considered to be less serious might have to go without professional medical care.

The newest form of delivering health care, telemedicine, has now taken up some of the slack caused by the lack of medical professionals. Computers and technology allow doctors to see patients without putting their own lives at risk. From the perspective of the medical profession telemedicine allows an expansion of the patient base, permits consultation with specialists in other locations and is cost effective, both for the patient and doctor. The latter point is especially relevant to patients who might have to travel for medical care. With telemedicine additional costs, such as travel, eating out, and lodging can be avoided.

Drawbacks to telemedicine are that it provides minimal examinations, the patient is not at the location where the testing is done, and different geographic or political locations have differing regulations. Additionally, if the internet fails during an examination the process might need to begin again.

Lastly, it should be noted that telemedicine might work best with people who have access to home technology and have the educational levels necessary to integrate the doctor's orders into their health care situation.

Pandemic resilience then begins with healthcare. Technology has created new healthcare opportunities but it is far from perfect. What the COVID-19 crisis has taught us is that there are no simple answers to a worldwide pandemic in which the number of patients is in the millions and medical facilities and personnel are strained to the limit.

25 QUESTIONS ABOUT HEALTH IN A PANDEMIC

The following questions are some of the questions that we might want to ask about our health during a pandemic. We provide what we consider to be sensible answers but we freely admit that we are not physicians, with whom you should consult before taking any action.

1. **How do we balance risk and health?**
   This question is not easy to answer. Risk is part

of life and all actions (or non-actions) involve risk. There is no such thing as a risk-free existence. The issue then is not how to avoid risk but rather how to keep risk to a minimum or to an acceptable level. Not seeing a medical professional for needed treatment is as risky (or may be riskier) than going to a medical office. Speak to the office manager, make sure that they know your situation and then follow the guidelines.

2. **What do I do if I think I am getting sick?**
   Getting sick is a broad term. Learn what the symptoms of the pandemic are. If you show manifestations, call your physician and go to the emergency room (if well enough to drive). Be sure to bring a mask with you and have a small packed bag with essentials, such as a toothbrush, and a change of underwear already packed. If you are not able to drive then call an ambulance and have the ambulance take you to the hospital. If you think you might be contagious then try to stay away from loved ones and other people whom you might infect.

3. **What books and medicines do I need to keep in case of an emergency and medical help is not available?**
   The following list is neither conclusive nor complete. It is meant only to get you started. The best thing to do is to create a list with your

personal physician. They will be familiar with your particular medical needs. If you cannot contact a physician or you do not have one, then the next best thing is to speak with a pharmacist and follow their guidelines. No home can be a full pharmacy but homes should have an assortment of medications, such as the following:

- Some form of pain reliever
- Some form of bandage and way to clean a wound
- Some form of hydrocortisone
- Something for diarrhea
- Some form of allergy relief medication
- An antacid
- Bacitracin or other antibiotic for minor skin injuries
- Some over-the-counter medicine for stomach upset
- Some form of antifungal medication

With regard to literature to be kept in the home consider books such as *The Mayo Clinic Book of Alternative Medicines and Home Remedies*. You might add to your library a book on herbal remedies and also a layperson's book on medications and pharmaceuticals. Again, it is best that you speak with your physician, healthcare provider and a pharmacist for their most up-to-date recommendations.

4. **What additional items should I have in my medical supply kit or medical chest?**

Each person is different and you should go over this list first with your physician and then with a pharmacist. Remember that all medications have expiration dates so it is a good idea to review medicines and other items in your medical chest on a regular basis (at least once a year). Legally dispose of expired medications and replace them. When storing medications it is a good idea to discuss the location with a pharmacist. For example, bathroom medical cabinets tend to be warmer and more humid than other locations in your home. Make sure that you understand the temperature range in which medications can be stored.

5. **What are my options for calling for help in case of a medical crisis?**

   Much depends on whom you know and where you are located. In most cases, if it's an emergency dialing 911 makes the most sense. The 911-dispatcher will determine if you need an ambulance. If it's not a question of life and death and you have a physician, get the physician's 24-hour number and keep it where everyone in your household can find it. It is also helpful to have in a visible location a list of any allergies you may have and all the medications you take. Finally there are a number of other emergency numbers that if needed can be called. Among these are:

- The poison control center
- The police and fire department
- Emergency number for a veterinarian

Have an emergency card that contains family names, dates of birth and special medical conditions. Assure that this emergency card is in at least one location where everyone in the household can find it during an emergency.

6. **What is the CDC and why are their guidelines important?**

The CDC (Center for Disease Control) is part of the United States Department of Health and Human Services. Its role is to protect the U.S. population from domestic and foreign health threats. It employs many of the nation's top medical experts and researchers, provides grants to universities, and informs the public on ways to stay healthy during public health crises, such as a pandemic.

The CDC has many of the world's top infectious disease specialists. It provides the most current data and suggestions on what to—or not to—do during a public health crisis. Following the CDC's guidelines helps you to protect your family and yourself.

7. **Who is most vulnerable during a pandemic?**

Different diseases and illnesses attack different groups of people. These cohorts might be due to age, gender, location or even race or ethnicity. Using COVID-19 as an example, this disease has been especially hard on older people. People with prior health conditions (especially lung conditions, cardiovascular disease, diabetes, chronic respiratory disease, and cancer are more likely to develop serious cases of COVID-19.

Of course, the less one is around other people the safer you are. People who must interact with others or enter into unprotected areas might also be at higher risk.

It's wise to stay regularly informed through a medical expert. It cannot be stated enough that information that appears to be true on any particular day may change as a health crisis evolves. This is especially true at the beginning of a pandemic.

8. **How important is having a personal relationship with a doctor or medical professional?**

Our body is a work of art and the more that a medical professional knows your particular body the better. Many people tend to forget that physicians are also human beings. Although they will try to treat all people in the most professional manner, humans tend to prioritize those people with whom they have a personal relationship.

9. **What is the difference between a physician assistant (PA) and a physician?**
A physician, often called simply a "doctor" in common parlance is a person who has gone through medical school and is proficient in diagnosing ailments and determining which treatments and medications are correct.

In the United States, after graduating with a B.A. or a B.S., a physician has an additional four years of medical schooling, plus three to seven years of "residency"—practical training for a specialty in a supervised medical facility. After a successful residency a U.S. physician must be nationally board certified and be licensed in the state where the physician is to practice medicine.

A physician assistant (PA) usually requires a four-year degree plus an additional 27 months of training, and at least one year of clinical rotation. PAs are required to take professional ongoing educational courses and retesting of their medical knowledge. PAs work under a physician's supervision and may assist in surgery but not perform it.

10. **What precautions should I take if I have to go into a doctor's office during a pandemic?**
Assuming this is a scheduled appointment the physician's office manager, nurse or secretary will inform you of the office's protocols. During

pandemics these may include the wearing of masks, waiting outside of the office, and payment only by non-touch means, such as a credit card.

Physicians' offices must follow state laws and protocols. If you have special medical needs be sure to discuss protective options before your visit.

11. **Should I avoid going to a dentist until the pandemic has subsided?**

The simple answer is no. Dental offices have taken extra measures to assure their patients' safety and their own. Prior to visiting the dentist, be sure to review with the office manager or dental nurse their office requirements during a time of pandemic and make sure that they are aware of any particular medical condition you may have.

12. **What foods should I take during a pandemic?**

Good nutrition is basic to staying healthy and fighting off illness. Drink lots of pure water. The Centers for Disease Control recommends eating foods that are high in Vitamin C and zinc ("Food and Coronavirus" par. 43). Other recommended foods are lean meats, fortified milk and milk alternatives, legumes, whole grains, nuts and seeds. By eating a variety of foods you cover a wide range of nutritional needs and achieve a well balanced diet.

13. **What vitamins are recommended to stay healthy?**

Consider the following foods that are rich in anti-viral vitamins:

- Vitamin A, found in oily fish, egg yokes, cheese, tofu, nuts and foods rich in beta-carotene such as carrots and pumpkins.
- B vitamins, found in such foods as green leafy vegetables, fruits, nuts and seeds, chicken and meats.
- Vitamin C, found in citric fruits such as oranges and lemons.
- Vitamin E, found in nuts, avocados, leafy green vegetables and natural vegetable oils.
- Vitamin D, gotten through limited exposure to the sun, but be careful not to burn or over expose yourself. Food sources for Vitamin D include eggs, fish and milk products that have been fortified with Vitamin D.

In addition to vitamins you need minerals. The three most important pandemic-fighting minerals are iron, zinc and selenium. Iron is found in meat, chicken and fish, whole grains and some breakfast cereals. Zinc is found in seafoods (especially oysters), meat, chicken, dried beans and nuts. Selenium is found in nuts (especially Brazil nuts), cereals and mushrooms.

Consult with either your physician or a nutritionist to determine what foods are best for you.

14. **Is it safe to exercise during a pandemic?**
There is no reason *not* to exercise during a pandemic. The issue is more a question of "where" rather than "if." If you are going to a gym, make sure that the gym uses proper precautions. The same applies to any other public space such as swimming pools and basketball courts. It is necessary to maintain a distance of about two meters (6 feet) from other people. If in close contact, wash your hands regularly and shower upon returning home.

Many people prefer to exercise alone and in a place where no other people are present. Wearing a mask and social distancing are not necessary when alone or far from others.

15. **What are two or three positive things that I can do for my health during a pandemic?**
These are simple: wash your hands for at least 20 seconds often, eat well balanced meals, drink plenty of fluids, especially pure water, and get at least seven hours of sleep each night. Remember that stress kills! So take things with a grain of salt and learn to smile.

16. **How important is sunlight and outdoor exercise?**
Sunlight and outdoor exercise is essential both for good physical and mental health. Lack of sunlight can cause depression, the

turning to drugs and alcohol, and even provoke a desire for physical isolation. Being outdoors allows us to breathe fresh air, and use our muscles.

17. **How much water should a person try to consume on a daily basis?**
    Our bodies are about 60% water. We lose water throughout the day through urination and sweating. Most health authorities recommend that we take in about two liters of water per day. Two liters are about a half a gallon, or eight full glasses of water. But this rule will vary according to individual body types, amount of exercise, climatic conditions, and weather. Remember too that many fruits and some vegetables contain high amounts of water. As a general rule, though, follow these three guidelines:
    - When thirsty, drink until you quench your thirst!
    - During periods when you sweat, such as in heat or during hard exercise, increase your fluids.
    - Ask your physician about the right quantities of water necessary for your body type, sex, physical location, age, and obesity issues you may have.

18. **Do we need more sleep during a pandemic?**

The short answer is yes. For example, in an article concerning COVID-19 and sleep published in *UChicago Medicine*, Lisa Medalie states that "Ample sleep supports the immune system, which reduces the risk of infection and can improve outcomes for people fighting a virus. On the other hand, sleep deprivation weakens the body's defense system and makes people more vulnerable to contracting a virus." The Sleep Foundation reinforces her words and notes that "Sleep is a critical biological process, and as we juggle the mental, physical, and emotional demands of the pandemic, it's arguably more important than ever" (Suni).

More to the point, about confronting the COVID-19 pandemic, sleep becomes even more essential because of its wide-ranging benefits for physical and mental health. The following points are among the many reasons why sleep is so important:

- "Sleep empowers an effective immune system. Solid nightly rest strengthens our body's defenses. Studies have even found that lack of sleep can make some vaccines less effective.
- "Sleep heightens brain function. Our mind works better when we get good sleep, contributing to complex thinking, learning, memory, and decision-making. For adults and children adapting to work and school at home, good sleep can help them stay sharp.

- "Sleep enhances mood. Lack of sleep can make a person irritable, drag down their energy level, and cause or worsen feelings of depression.
- "Sleep improves mental health. Besides depression, studies have found that a lack of sleep is linked with mental health conditions like anxiety disorder, bipolar disorder, and Post-Traumatic Stress Disorder (PTSD).

"Experts agree that getting consistent, high-quality sleep improves virtually all aspects of health, which is why it is worthy of our attention during the coronavirus pandemic" (Suni).

As a rule of thumb consider that children ages 6–13 need between 9–11 hours of sleep, teenagers between 8–10 hours of sleep, adults (18–64 years old) between 7–9 hours of sleep, and adults older than 64 need between 7–8 hours of sleep per night (Van Kyk).

19. **What are healthy sleep patterns for children during a pandemic?**

Children need 10–11 hours of regenerative sleep time per day during a pandemic. Less time than this can cause symptoms of tiredness, lack of attention, or a weakened immune system. On the *Rise and Shine* website of Children's National, Daniel Lewin writes that "Sleep deprivation and sleeping at the wrong time of the 24 hour day can harm a child's developing brain, and drowsiness can affect a child's school performance. Inadequate sleep can also result in bad moods and weakened immune systems."

Experts recommend that children have established bedtimes and that parents stick to this routine. It's also recommended that electronics be turned off at least one hour prior to bedtimes. Parents should discuss sleeping habits and needs with the child's pediatrician and the pediatrician should be updated on any problems or irregularities that a parent might observe.

20. What are the different types of face masks and which are best?

Many states and localities now require the use of face masks when a person is outside or in an enclosed space with other people. In July of 2020 this policy was endorsed by both the U.S. Centers for Disease Control (CDC) and the World Health Organization (WHO). Currently there are three types of masks in use: surgical masks, respirator type masks such as N95 or FFP2, and cloth face coverings.

Surgical masks are meant to be single use masks, and loosely fit over the nose and mouth. They function well against large droplets from coughs or sneezes, but not against smaller droplets or particles like coronavirus.

N95 or FFP2 masks fit closely to the face and form seals around the mouth and nose. They filter out pathogens from the air. These are believed to be the most effective masks.

Cloth masks come in a variety of colors and shapes. The most effective ones are made of tightly woven cotton fabrics, but they are less effective than the N95 variety.

21. **How do I wear a face mask safely?**

The CDC provides the following guidelines for wearing cloth face coverings ("How to"):

- Wash your hands before putting on your face covering.
- Place it over your nose and mouth and secure it under your chin.
- Fit it as snugly as possible against the sides of your face.
- Make sure you can breathe easily.

The CDC's guidelines remind us of two good reasons for wearing proper face masks:

- Protect others in case you're infected with COVID-19 but don't have symptoms.
- Protect yourself from infection in public settings when around people who don't live in your household, especially if it's difficult for you to distance yourself from others by at least six feet.
- Wear a face covering correctly for maximum protection. Wear it over your mouth and nose, not around your neck or up on your forehead.
- Don't touch the face covering. If you do, wash your hands or use hand sanitizer to disinfect.

22. **Can I reuse a disposable face mask?**
Most people know that cloth face masks can be washed and cared for just as you might care for any other intimate garment. Many people ask if disposable face masks are for use just one time or if they can they be used multiple times.

The CDC gives us some common sense advice about this. It states that a disposable face mask can be reused if you do not touch your mask, or if you wash your hands with soap and water prior to touching the mask.

What is known now is that the COVID-19 virus cannot normally survive outside a host for longer than 48 hours. So, a mask can be reused if it's stored isolated somewhere for 24-48 hours, which most likely renders it virus free. But do not reuse a mask that is visibly dirty, soiled or torn. The best practice is to rotate a small supply of face masks so that no single mask is reused within a 48-hour period (Breen).

23. **What precautions should I use when riding on public transportation?**
Public transportation falls into a number of sub categories:
- Air transportation
- Public surface mass transit such as buses and trains
- Single-usage transportation such as taxis or car services

Airlines have taken extra precautions to assure traveler safety. The have installed new air filtration systems, food and beverages are served in closed containers and in many cases both onboard airline personnel and passengers are required to wear masks.

The situation is less certain within an airport terminal. In reality, any terminal—bus, train, maritime or air—exposes the person to less than adequate social distancing.

There is no one answer to this question as is made clear in a *New York Times* article by Jane Levere. She sums up the situation when she states that "As to the airports, they are screening passengers' temperatures through high- and low-tech means; using biometric screening to speed check-in, security and customs and immigration processes; and using autonomous robots to clean terminal floors. But none of it is consistent. And it's unclear whether the measures are enough."

24. How does a pandemic affect mental health?

There is little doubt that pandemics are not only hard on the body but also on our minds. According to the CDC ("Coping") some of the things that cause mental anguish and, therefore, increased anxiety, are:

- Fear and worry about our health and the health of loved ones, our financial situation or job, or loss of support services
- Changes in sleep or eating patterns
- Difficulty sleeping or concentrating
- Worsening of chronic health problems
- Worsening of mental health conditions
- Increased use of tobacco, alcohol and other substances

25. **How can I lower my stress and anxiety during a pandemic?**

Pandemics are not an easy time, and when we are worried about our families and our finances, we are forced to stay at home, and suffer a change of routine, the situation becomes even more difficult. There's one first rule of thumb to follow: "do not lose your dignity." That means get dressed, maintain good hygiene and proper grooming, establish a daily schedule, and eat regular, well-balanced meals. Make lists of what you want to accomplish each day, and exercise at regularly. In other words, do everything possible to maintain a state of normalcy during a period of abnormality.

Writing in the *Psychology Today* journal, David Braucher underscores these principles when he advises to "Stick with Old Routines as Much as Possible":

- "Do what makes us feel like ourselves. When possible, we should try to keep our old routines. For example: If taking a shower and getting dressed for work in the morning is important to feeling like ourselves, we should get dressed for work even if we are working remotely and no one will see us.
- "Keep to the schedule. Maintain the same schedule we had before the crisis. For example: If we used to work out after work, once our remote workday is over, we can do an online workout.
- "Workarounds. The internet is abuzz with workarounds from 'FaceTime dates' to 'virtual happy hours' with coworkers over video chat...."

Our old routines are important, but we can also make new routines for ourselves, such as the following:

- "Make a new schedule. If our old schedules don't work, we need to make new ones and stick to them.
- "Do what makes us feel effective. In times like these when we don't feel like we have many choices, it's imperative that we do things that make us feel effective—a great antidote to any sense of futility and helplessness. An instructor at a senior center calls her students to see how they are doing, giving her a sense of being useful. 'I felt more like myself. That's what I do, I connect with people.'

- "Do the things you never had time for. Over the years, many of us have found ourselves wishing we had more time in our day. Now, we may feel we have too much. This too will come to an end. Use the extra time to read a book or spend time with your family, even if just on the phone. Treat this time as a valuable gift. It will soon be gone."

▪ ▪ ▪

We wrote this chapter at the height of the pandemic. It was a time of uncertainty and confusion. As the COVID-19 pandemic developed it became clear that this chapter's information is not only correct but will be useful when another pandemic occurs in the future.

Its theme is that, during a pandemic, taking care of oneself is a moral obligation not only to yourself but also to those whom you love. The questions asked and answered above all point to the fact that good health starts with the basics: eating well, good hygiene, and getting proper rest and exercise.

This chapter also teaches us that pandemics are dynamic and not static. Conditions change and sometimes medical experts need to update their advice. What does not change, however, is that each of us needs to have an ongoing relationship with a medical professional whom we trust and that each of us is responsible not only for our own health but also for our actions that impact the lives of others.

CHAPTER

3

KEEPING HIGH SPIRITS

JUST AS HEALTH defines our "outer being" so does spirituality define our "inner being." We can measure our health, take our blood pressure and listen to the beat of the heart. The same is not true of spiritual health. Our spiritual health is unique to each of us and is beyond statistical measurement.

INCONVENIENCES AND SUFFERING

Although a healthy spirit will not prevent all forms of disease, an unhealthy spirit might well increase the likelihood of illness. When writing in the U.S. National Library of Medicine journal about coping with suffering, Christina Puchalski highlighted Victor Frankl's own words about his experience in a Nazi concentration camp, that "Man is not destroyed by suffering; he is destroyed by suffering without meaning."

One of the challenges physicians face is to help people find meaning and acceptance in the midst of suffering and chronic illness. Medical ethicists have reminded us that religion and spirituality form the basis of meaning and purpose for many people (Delagran).

At the same time, while patients struggle with the physical aspects of their disease, they have other pain as well: pain related to mental and spiritual suffering, to an inability to engage the deepest questions of life.

WHAT IS SPIRITUALITY?

In some sense spirituality is the other side of the coin from physical health. As we saw in chapter "2", physical health is somewhat akin to chemistry; it follows a formula and has exact do's and don't's. Often physical health is objective in nature. We know scientifically that smoking is bad for our lungs and that eating healthy fruits and vegetables are good for the body.

In that sense, spirituality is the opposite. It is not objective but subjective knowledge. There are no spirituality formulas and what might be a spiritual experience for one person may not be so for the next.

Despite this fact, most people have a sense of the intangible that permeates through their lives. We might call this intangible our spiritual, or our artistic side, or our emotional side. It is the effect that a piece of music or art might have on us, the viewing of a beautiful moment or an intimate moment with someone or something. Thus, spirituality is ubiquitous yet indefinite; it can be a constant or a fleeting moment.

Just as in the case of the physical, spirituality too is necessary; and during a pandemic our spiritual sides play an essential role in how we cope with ourselves, with the world around us and with others.

"Spirituality is … a sense of connection to something bigger than each of us, and it typically involves a search for meaning in life."

In many ways the physical and the spiritual connect. Many have come to ask if a healthy spirit is not part of a person's overall health. Despite the connections between a healthy body, a healthy spirit, and a healthy psyche, too many of us do everything possible to avoid dealing with all aspects of this triangle of life.

How many of us neither know nor want to know the inner parts of our life? Some people spend their lifetime seeking to hide themselves from themselves. Self-knowledge can scare us. But during a pandemic, when we might spend hours alone, we can gain such inner knowledge through what we now call euphemistically "shelter-in-place." It's during such times that we might well learn that we cannot hide from ourselves.

The word "spirituality" may mean different things to different people. Dictionary definitions of it are rarely adequate. For example, the Merriam-Webster dictionary of the American language defines *spirituality* as "1: something that in ecclesiastical law belongs to the church or to a cleric as such; 2: clergy; 3: sensitivity or attachment to religious values; 4: the quality or state of being spiritual."

Another, perhaps better, definition of spirituality comes from the University of Minnesota's Health Center's webpage when it tells us that "Spirituality is a broad concept with room for many perspectives. In general, it includes a sense of connection to something bigger than each of us, and it typically involves a search for meaning in life. As such, it is a universal human experience—something that touches us all. People may describe a spiritual experience as sacred or transcendent or simply a deep sense of aliveness and interconnectedness" (Delegran).

What might be a spiritual experience for one person might not be for another person. Like the viewing of art, or the tasting of food, our sense of spirituality is unique to each of us. Spirituality cannot be described, only felt, and to be spiritual is to go beyond words and enter into the realm of the "what is but cannot be." A spiritual person asks questions such as—

What is my place in the universe?

What is the meaning of life?

What is the meaning of my life?

How do I make moral decisions?

Are we merely intelligent animals?

Do we exist for a purpose beyond ourselves?

Although these questions are universal, none of us necessarily comes to the same conclusion or has the same answers. The questions are universal but the answers are personal.

These answers touch the very basis of our being, and as such each person's answer will reflect his or her uniqueness. Indeed, one of the things that distinguishes us from other forms of life is that we ask reflexive questions like these.

Many of these questions are both spiritual and religious. In the western world, at times religion and spirituality overlap and both intersect with mysticism, psychology and physics. For purposes of this book, however, we shall distinguish between the latter two, not out of lack of respect for religion or mysticism, but because this book is meant to be open to everyone; people of all faiths or of no faith, people who see the world through western eyes and those who see the world through a different lens.

25 QUESTIONS TO EXPLORE SPIRITUALITY

This chapter concludes with 25 questions that explore spirituality in general and during pandemic times. Not that pandemics require any different approach to spirituality, but pandemics, like all prolonged crises, certainly tax our beings beyond normal times and give us good reasons for extraordinary introspection.

1. **What is (a) the spirit?**
   This might be the most difficult of all questions. Different peoples, religions and cultures have different interpretations of what the "spirit" is. All too often we make the mistake of assuming "what I think is what you think." To add to our difficulties most people are not sure they really know what the word means. A good exercise is to ask yourself this very question and then to write out your answer. Compare your answer with that found in the dictionary, the guidance that your own faith gives you and what other faiths have to say. In this way you can begin to define the term for yourself and see how your definition impacts the way you live and interact with others.

2. **Is the spirit the same as the soul?**
The answer to this question depends on the religious tradition to which you adhere. Not only is the word "spirit" hard to define but also the word "soul" is even harder to define. Each religious tradition has its own interpretation of this word. Even within the mainstream religious traditions there are multiple variations. To add to the difficulty of defining the word soul, the word is laced with both linguistic and religious nuances. Some people clearly believe that there is no such thing as a soul, others firmly believe that the soul is the very source from which life springs forth. A time of pandemic is a time when there are many opportunities for reflective thinking and personal study. This could be a time to go beyond yourself and to explore the deeper meaning of words such as the spirit and the soul.

3. **Is a personal sense of spirituality the same as the classical western idea of spirituality?**
Each person's sense of the spiritual might be different. The famous early 20th century philosopher Martin Buber in his classic work *I and Thou* shows how a person finds spirituality even in a relationship with a tree. During a time of pandemics when scientific knowledge is often in flux (good science is never settled science, so good science is always a bit in flux) it is essen-

tial that each person learn to relate to those indefinable parts of life we call "the spirit" and seek not canned answers but personal answers that come from the interrelationship of the inner depths of that person with the world in which we live.

4. **Can I be spiritual and not religious?**
   The short answer is yes. There are many people who claim to be spiritual but not religious. By that they usually mean that they have rejected the outer tenants of a particular faith.

5. **Do different people define spirituality in different ways?**
   Yes, no two people have the same sense of the spiritual. Each person is a unique being and each person sees the world through very different eyes.

6. **Do religion and spirituality overlap?**
   They overlap but are not the same. One can be spiritual and not religious or religious and not spiritual. Religions are usually a set of organized beliefs and practices and these beliefs and practices tend to be shared by a particular group. Spirituality is personal and transitory. One can have moments of spirituality. Religious principles can be taught, but spirituality is usually personal and comes from within.

7. **Is prayer the way to express spirituality?**
No, spirituality can be expressed through multiple means such as prayer, the fine arts, an appreciation of nature, a sense of community or the observation of a particular or singular event in the natural world. Spirituality, as different from religion, is personal; each person may have his or her own spiritual experience.

8. **How do I hear the inner voice that resonates from the depth of my being?**
As related in the Bible, the prophet Elijah hears within himself the "still small voice"—"the sound of silence" (1 Kings 19:13). This literary allusion has intrigued humans at least from Biblical times. Can we hear silence? Is there an inner sense that speaks to us without words? This question is based on the assumption that the person believes that a human being has a soul.

During a pandemic, when there might be feelings of isolation, learning to hear one's soul (or gut or inner wisdom) might be more critical than ever.

To hear the still small voice of our inner self is neither easy nor simple but that voice might allow us the resilience to face the unknown with confidence and a sense of hope. during a pandemic.

9. **To be spiritual must one withdraw from the world?**

There are certainly those who do withdraw from the world around them in order to pursue spirituality. There are religious communities within major religions such as Catholicism or Buddhism, where some of their members have left the world of the secular so as to be unencumbered by their spiritual pursuits.

Even in these religions, though, one can be spiritual and still be active in society. Other cultural and religious communities reject the idea that to be spiritual one must be removed from society and argue that spirituality is found in the intersection of the personal and the social. Thus for them spirituality comes from one's active role in society.

10. Is work a form of spirituality?

Another way that we express our spirituality is through work. Work shouldn't be a dirty word; it is not something to be avoided. Rather, work is a way to define our humanity. Genesis speaks of Adam (2:15) as working. Work is not punishment but the chance to explore our creativity. Note that we are not only commanded to rest on the seventh day but also to work on the other six days of the week.

Work can be viewed as a form of prayer. It can be nothing more than a way to earn one's keep or it can be used to take us to a greater meaning, to become "fixers of the world," to make the world a better place.

Not only do we work to earn money, but also the spiritual person works toward self-improvement. To work, to struggle with oneself is a form of prayer. It is the essence of defining who we are and what we are about. To work symbolizes that no one in this world owes us anything, that we have been given capabilities and opportunities and it is for us to use them or to lose them. The spiritual person knows that the choice is his or hers.

11. **How does spirituality take us from a sense of obligation to a sense of opportunity?**

Donald Walsch in his book *Conversations with God* writes that "Opportunity, not obligation, is the cornerstone of religion, the basis of all spirituality. So long as you see it the other way around, you will have missed the point. Relationship—your relationship to all things—was created as your perfect tool in the work of the soul. That is why all human relationships are sacred ground. It is why every personal relationship is holy." (Walsch 137–138.)

What Walsch argues is that spirituality is more than a mere moment of "nirvana." It is the hard work of interacting with those around us.

During a pandemic we have the opportunity to improve our relationships and deepen them. When we are under some form of quarantine we have the chance to know the others in our family circle in new and creative ways.

12. **How do we define lost opportunities?**
If we see spirituality as an opportunity to interact with those we love then we can ask this question: Are our relationships windows into the depths of our souls? If so, what do you see through your window? Think about the impact of your spiritual assumptions on the way you do business and handle money. In regards to the law, do you have the sense that the world was created only for your sake? Do laws exist only for others or for those too stupid to learn how to get around them? Are you passionate about your work, family, friends, and significant other? Do you see work and food as only a means to survive or do you relish life, and get the most out of each day?

Most religions have a word for breaking their law: "sin." Biblical Hebrew, however, does not see sin as a transgression against God but rather as a lost opportunity. In Hebrew the translation of the verb *sin* is a concept that means to "miss the mark," to "lose an opportunity."

13. **What is prayer?**
The fairest answer to this question is to state that there is no one correct answer. For example, to pray in English is derived from the Vulgate Latin word "precare" meaning to

ask earnestly, to beg or to entreat. In Hebrew, on the other hand, to pray is to engage in a self-struggle or self-judgment. Prayer is often divided into the following four subcategories:

- Formal community prayer
- Informal community prayer
- Formal personal prayer
- Informal personal prayer

Formal prayers are those that are prescribed by a religion or faith group. These prayers are written down and recited word for word. A person can say prayers as part of a religious service (community prayer) or as an individual. In both cases they are formalist in nature, and they reinforce specific beliefs and ideologies. Informal prayer might be closer to spirituality as it comes from the person rather than the group. It expresses a personal relationship to a power higher than oneself. Informal prayers may take place within a formalized service or outside of a religious setting.

14. **Is prayer a part of spirituality?**

This answer depends on how one defines prayer. If we are speaking about formal and set prayer then the answer is closer to no than to yes. If we are speaking about personal prayer then the answer is closer to yes than to no. Furthermore different religions, faith grouping, or ethnic groups have different understandings of the word prayer. English tends to use a Christianized version of the word. In other languages such as Hebrew, Hindi, or Japanese the word for prayer has a different connotation and sentiment.

15. **Does spirituality lead to ethical behavior?**
Spirituality is outside of the realm of ethics. Because spirituality is personal, it might lead to a sense of what's ethical, but that's a spurious outcome rather than consequential.

16. **What is ethical behavior?**
The word *ethics* has multiple nuances. Accountants in training through the online My Accounting Course website are taught that "An ethical behavior is the application of moral principles in a given situation. It means to behave according to the moral standards set by the society which we live in."

Often we see the study of ethics combined with different professions. When dealing with the workplace, for example, William Mahan of the *Work Institute* states that "Ethics in the workplace is defined as the moral code that guides the behavior of employees with respect to what is right and wrong in regard to conduct and decision making. Ethical decision making in the workplace takes into account the individual employee's best interest and also takes into account the best interest of those impacted...[and] the organization itself should exemplify standards of ethical conduct."

Among the professions with a great need for strong ethics is medicine where life and death decisions are made routinely.

17. **What are the Noahide laws and what purpose do they serve?**

As discussed in question 8, there's a gap between what is considered ethical, legal, and universally right. One attempt to create a universal standard—no matter what a culture might determine to be ethical—is called the Noahide laws. The New World Encyclopedia has this: "According to Jewish tradition, the Noahide Laws...refer to seven religious laws that...are considered to be morally binding on non-Jews. These laws are listed in the Talmud and elucidated by post-Talmudic authorities." These "laws" are found in at least three parts of the Talmudic writings and are meant to define universal morality, versus Jewish morality, as follows:

- Not to worship idols
- Not to curse God
- To establish courts of justice
- Not to commit murder/participate in bloodshed/or rob
- Not to commit adultery, bestiality or other acts of sexual immorality
- Not to eat the flesh of a living animal

18. **How are law and ethics different?**

Although we hope that laws are also ethical, they may not be and at times these two important concepts might even be opposed to one another. On the whole, laws are principles set down by governments. They may reflect ethics or not, although for a law to exist it must have at least the passive acceptance of the majority of the population it governs. Hypothetically laws live within time while ethics live outside of time.

The case of medical and recreational marijuana is an example of this. It's now legal in many places to use marijuana for recreational or medical purposes. And while medical use may be considered legal and ethical, the recreational use may be illegal.

19. **Can a sense of religion, spirituality, or law help me to grow as a person?**

Yes and no. Many people find that both religion and spirituality force them to ask profound questions regarding some of life's basic questions: What is life? What is my purpose in life? Is there life after death? Why does a loving God permit evil to exist? Others find such "wisdom" to be more dogma than soul-searching. Much depends on the person.

Law rarely serves to make us better people. Rather, it permits guidelines to keep from creating serious problems for ourselves and for others.

The American system is based on rights.

Human beings, by nature of their birth, are accorded specific rights. And then there are systems that are based not on rights but on duties, like the duty of a person to not commit murder.

20. **Can spirituality substitute for human contact?**
No, we need other humans. Technology helps and we now have electronic parties via social media platforms, but humans are social animals and as such nothing replaces other human beings. In the journal *Psychology Today* Elliot Cohen states this fact plainly when he writes that "According to Aristotle, human beings are 'social animals' " and therefore naturally seek the companionship of others as part of their well being . . . This human social dynamic includes building and maintaining intimate or close social relationships."

21. **How do I use a sense of spirituality to help get me through being isolated during a pandemic?**
Human beings are social animals; we need each other. Few human beings choose to be hermits, and one of the worst punishments that a human being can receive in prison is to be placed in solitary confinement.

This need for the other is one of the reasons that the shelter-in-place policies have been so hard on those living alone, especially the elderly. One way to survive this trauma is to connect to something other than oneself. Some do this by practicing yoga, others through meditation and prayer, still others by becoming television or film junkies. For some a sense of spirituality connects us to ideas and concepts beyond ourselves.

22. **Does spirituality help explain why bad things happen?**

Spirituality differs from religion in this regard. Spirituality, however, does not seek to answer "why" questions. Just as social scientists avoid the *why* and focus only on the when, where, what, who and how of events, *why* questions are not a part of spirituality. On the other hand, many religions seek to provide answers to why questions such as: Why is there evil in the universe? Why did God create the world, humanity or even me? Said in another way: why do bad things happen to good people?

23. **Does finding a purpose in one's life help to order the world in which we live?**

Life is chaotic and science teaches us that entropy—that all order eventually breaks down and becomes chaotic—is an ever-present phenomenon. The laws of entropy argue that nothing is forever; all things physical pass away. The Bible tends to see God as the opposite of entropy; that is, that God brings order from chaos rather than chaos from order.

This tension between order and chaos is also a part of our lives. During periods of pandemic we are faced with issues of the unknown, and although we may clean and organize our homes, all too often our lives feel as if they are in shambles.

For some a connection with forces stronger than themselves helps to unite the person with a reversal of entropy. In that sense, spirituality might connect the person to being a part of something greater than themselves and permit a mental ordering of the person's particular reality.

24. **Are animals spiritual?**

The answer to this question might depend on about which animals we are speaking. For example, Barbara King writes in *The Atlantic* about Jane Goodall's famous work with chimpanzees in Tanzania. Goodall described how she watched a group of chimpanzees transcend from a boisterous episode to quiescence as the troop settled together to watch a waterfall, "'perhaps triggered by feelings of awe, wonder' for magnificent natural features or events. Chimpanzees are so similar to us, she asks, 'Why wouldn't they also have feelings of some kind of spirituality?' "

In her *Atlantic* article, King also writes that in

his book *Religious Affects: Animality, Evolution, and Power*, Donovan Schaefer, an Oxford University lecturer, "rejects the Euro-American tendency to equate religion with belief, text, and language. Religion is something we feel in and express with our whole bodies, Schaefer insists, and once we realize this, we are free to see religion in other animals in certain instances of their embodied and emotional practices."

Steven Kotler in *Psychology Today* also grapples with the idea that animals might be either spiritual or even religious. He argues that "For now, let's keep the door open to the idea that animals can be spiritual beings and let's consider the evidence for such a claim. Meager as it is, available evidence says 'Yes, animals can have spiritual experiences' and we need to conduct further research and engage in interdisciplinary discussions before we say that animals cannot and do not experience spirituality."

25. **How do I translate spirituality into actions?**

If spirituality is just a fleeting moment then it cannot be translated into action, but if spirituality is a lifestyle or a series of actionable beliefs then it can very much become action.

People like Mother Teresa took the spiritual and transformed belief into living realities. Many Jews incorporate the *mitzvah* system into their daily lives, seeking to perform *tikun olam*—the fixing of a broken world by acts of good deeds and loving kindness. Actionable spirituality is often translated via a religious community, but there are people who live outside of standard religious communities and are called to act due to a sense of spirituality. Often political activists act from a sense of spirituality. We can sense a spiritual plane alongside a political plane in speeches of former presidents, such as John Kennedy.

■ ■ ■

Spirituality has many faces. It is hard to define and even harder to transfer from one person to another. As such in a time of pandemics our own sense of who we are, where we fit into the universe, and how we learn to become comfortable with ourselves is a basic tool of pandemic survival.

The good news is that our spirituality does not come from a book or a video; rather, our spirituality comes from within ourselves. It is a natural resource that money cannot buy.

People who find their purpose in the world and have an inner sense of self are wealthy persons no matter what their assets might be. Spirituality is the inner peace that fills the emptiness found within each of us, especially in trying times of isolation.

CHAPTER

4

SOCIAL ISSUES OF A PANDEMIC

LIVING THROUGH A pandemic alone, in social isolation, or with a set group of people, such as a family, is not easy. Non-stop togetherness, no matter how much one loves family, also has its challenges. During pandemics many couples not only argue, but their children also feel the anger, fear and frustration.

Family problems are felt not only in the U.S. but throughout the world. Thus, Yi-Ling Liu writing about China for the British Broadcasting Company (BBC) said that "Most notably the high-pressure environment of confinement, combined with the financial stress brought about by a COVID-19 burdened economy, has led to a rise in marital conflict, according to Susanne Choi, a sociologist at the Chinese University of Hong Kong."

Her findings are also reflected in the United States. According to a CNBC report (StatesAttorney.org), "More time spent together in quarantine can put added strain on (a couple's) relationships, especially those where problems already exist, and push the divorce rate up as a result. For couples with underlying problems, being confined to one space with the other person could theoretically expedite a divorce."

CONTRADICTIONS OF TOGETHERNESS

Arguments and disagreements between parents can be a common, unfortunate event. This characterizes many households and provokes pain and distress in many children even in normal circumstances, but it is highlighted even more in pandemic times.

Living together is never easy but when we lack personal time and space it becomes at best a challenge and at times destructive.

In reality, during "more normative times" most people in a family live parallel lives. We eat dinner together and might spend some family time together but we also find ways to maintain our own personal space and time.

The COVID-19 pandemic changed that reality, especially for those who have small or inadequate living quarters or for those whose family structure was wobbly even before the pandemic hit.

FORCED CONFINEMENT IS A STRESSOR

The number of social problems created by forced confinement can seem limitless. Parents who were still working found themselves seeking a quiet place to work. Children, deprived of friends and social interaction, became bored or grumpy. Grandparents and the elderly felt isolated from friends and family. Perhaps only our pets were pleased with the additional attention they received.

Distance Learning and Remote Work

During times of a pandemic, parents, many of whom are ill prepared for new roles, discovered that they were now running in-home classrooms, daycare centers, and creating at-home summer camps. Parents became counselors, cooks, home cleaners, and repair-persons. Many people, however, lack the skills and patience to be all of the above.

Space even in a large home is often limited and during periods of confinement personal space soon becomes a thing of the past. Children living in apartments or in large or less well-off families disproportionately suffered along with their parents. During a pandemic many children have little space in which to be a child, to run wild and to develop an inner sense of being.

Technology helps, however, even in homes fortunate enough to have one or more computers, and adequate living space, there is still a technology deficit. For example, we have learned that distance learning at best is a poor substitute for in-person classroom instruction, and provides almost no opportunities for socialization and playtime.

In reality most families, and especially poorer families, do not have adequate technological resources. This resource deficit often means that work-from-home scenarios puts a family into a state of conflict as both parents and children compete for computer time, if they have even one. It is not uncommon for work hours to collide with school hours. Thus, working parents might have need of the family's sole computer at the exact same time that children need to be on line at the same time for distance learning classes.

It should be emphasized that the above problems reflect the frustrations of middle and upper class families. In poorer families the situation can

---

> "… 'Many victims find themselves isolated in violent homes, without access to resources or friend or family networks'.… [and now] we are learning that due to schools being closed children that suffer from mental and physical abuse had no one else to whom to turn."

---

be much worse. In too many cases children have been reduced to distance-education that is "distance-learning" in name only. Many simply do not show up for on-line classes or fail to do assignments. As Kevin Huffman wrote in the *Washington Post*, "Poorer children don't just have less access to technology; they're also more likely to be home alone, because their parents do not have the privilege to telework during the quarantine. As Sarah Carpenter, executive director of the Memphis Lift, a parent advocacy organization, puts it: 'The lady next door has seven kids and no computers. The family up the street has no Internet. I'm afraid some families aren't going to do anything because some families simply can't do anything.'."

Even in the best of circumstances not only did children have to compete with working parents for computer time, but many families might not have been able to handle children of different age levels needing the same computers for distance learning, or simply needing personal attention, at the same time.

To add to life's extra problems due to a pandemic, many parents do not know how to be multi-subject teachers and tutors. To the credit of the teaching profession, and many school systems, educators recognized these problems almost from the start of the pandemic and many educational professionals did all that was possible to mitigate these problems.

Pandemics and Domestic Violence

Prior to COVID-19 few families had considered or were prepared for such a new situation. The result of this lack of preparedness was additional family frustrations and friction. We now know that family stress (along with both child and spousal abuse) has increased for many. Writing for *USA Today*, Candy Woodall quoted Dr. Norrell Atkinson, section chief of the child protection program at St. Christopher's Hospital for Children in Philadelphia as saying that "There are lots of stressors already.... The pandemic has put additional stress on every single family. That can certainly create a stressed-out parent, which can lead to abuse."

The forced stay-at-home regulations might also be responsible, at least in part, for an increase in family violence. For example, a May 2020 report by the Council of Foreign Relations (Bettinger-Lopez) reported that "Today, rising numbers of sick people, growing unemployment, increased anxiety and financial stress, and a scarcity of community resources have set the stage for an exacerbated domestic violence crisis. Many victims find themselves isolated in violent homes, without access to resources or friend and family networks. Abusers could experience heightened financial pressures and stress, increase their consumption of alcohol or drugs, and purchase or hoard guns as an emergency measure. Experts have characterized an 'invisible pandemic' of domestic violence during the COVID-19 crisis as a 'ticking time bomb' or a 'perfect storm'."

When economic hardships that families might be experiencing were combined with child-abuse issues, the situation for some became explosive. Elisabetta de Cao of the London School of Economics and Malte Sandner of the Institute for Employment Research wrote that "Economic hardship is considered a strong predictor of child abuse and neglect. [According to research by Jason] Lindo et al . . . *abuse and neglect* cases *decrease* by 7–8% when male employment *increases* by one percentage point, while such cases *increase* by 8–12% when female employment *increases* by one percentage point. A potential channel for these findings is the time spent with children. [In another research project, Dan] Brown and De Cao...estimate[d]

"... *abuse and neglect* cases *decrease* by 7–8% when male employment *increases* by one percentage point, while such cases *increase* by 8-12% when female employment *increases* by one percentage point.... [Researchers] estimate that a one percentage point increase in the unemployment rate leads to a 20% increase in neglect."

---

that a one percentage point increase in the unemployment rate leads to a 20% increase in neglect" (italics added).

As to be expected, the situation for the poor is much more precarious than for those who are economically more fortunate. The United Nations report (UN "Everyone Included" pars. 13–14) on the pandemic's impact on young people underlined this fact thus: "In terms of employment, youth are disproportionately unemployed, and those who are employed often work in the informal economy or gig economy, on precarious contracts or in the service sectors of the economy, that are likely to be severely affected by COVID-19. More than one billion youth are now no longer physically in school after the closure of schools and universities across many jurisdictions. The disruption in education and learning could have medium and long-term consequences on the quality of education, though the efforts made by teachers, school administrations, local and national governments to cope with the unprecedented circumstances to the best of their ability should be recognized."

Virtual Social Interaction Helps But Falls Short

There are countless other reasons why children might suffer from shelter-in-place policies. Youngsters are less emotionally able to handle long hours without going outside or seeing friends. Younger children may be emotionally damaged due to their parents' frustrations, anger, and fears. Families worry that resources that were once readily available have disappeared. Furthermore we are learning that due to schools being closed children that suffer from mental and physical abuse had no one else to whom to turn.

During the periods of isolation caused by a pandemic, computers also become major tools of social interaction. It has been via computers that everything from business meetings to children's birthday parties became "virtual" experiences. Poorer children, often not having any computer access or limited computer access and living in tight quarters, experienced even greater interpersonal frustrations along with social and learning setbacks.

To add to family frustrations and social challenges, the pandemic caused millions of people to be out of work, creating an economic situation that was dire at best. Parents had to worry about how they would provide food and shelter without an income.

As we shall see in chapter 4, there are millions of people in the United States and other parts of the world who live, or have been living, on a paycheck-to-paycheck or hand-to-mouth basis. Now in a period of layoffs middle class families have joined poorer families in not only having lost their income but in many cases their self-respect.

LONG-TERM EDUCATIONAL CONSEQUENCES

Not only do youths-at-risk suffer during a pandemic but even children in more privileged settings suffer. The world's educational system has had to adapt to lack of in-schooling education. Teachers have had to work under difficult circumstances and children of all social strata have had to adjust, along with their families, to new and often trying realities.

Pandemic Effects on Schools

As we might expect the closing of schools disproportionately impacts poor or disadvantaged children, many of whom also depended on school systems to provide basic nutrition and life skills. Many of these children may have parents who cannot provide either in-person learning aids or technical equipment necessary for distance learning.

The closing of schools has also resulted in the loss of extra curricular activities and learning. These activities are important learning situations for children of all ages and tend to aid social and physical growth. They are a necessary part of learning and filled in developmental voids from sports to the arts.

The fact that schools are closed also means that opportunities for semi-formal educational enhancement activities were no longer available either especially for underprivileged children. A United Nations report continues by stating that "With protracted closures, it will become a challenge to ensure that students return to school once reopened. To alleviate the situation, governments should ensure there is continuity in learning by promoting high-tech, low-tech and no-tech solutions, focusing in particular on reaching vulnerable groups. In addition, international cooperation to share best practices on effective responses will be instrumental" (UN "COVID-19 and Youth" 3).

Pandemic Effects on Higher Education

The isolation and closures due to the pandemic also impacted university students and faculty members. Non-commuting students did not know whether they needed to rent apartments or remain at their parents' home. Faculty members were not sure what types of lectures to prepare or how in-lab learning was to take place when students were not in the lab. Additionally, many universities have quasi-professional sports teams. For many university sports programs it is the football program that brings in the necessary funding to allow all other athletic activities to occur, and athletic teams are also a large part of a university's fundraising efforts.

The COVID-19 pandemic has forced the cancellation of multiple athletic events. Zac Al-Kateeb wrote in *U.S. Sporting News* that "The spread of the coronavirus (COVID-19) in the U.S. has forced college football decision-makers into a previously unthinkable choice: Whether to play this fall, or postpone the season. Those looming choices have reached a fever pitch in recent days, with the Big Ten and Pac-12 announcing on Tuesday they would cancel their respective fall seasons in favor of a spring campaign."

As many of these teams are located in "College towns" who receive a great deal of their tourism from football game attendees, cancellations impact not only the players but the communities' economic health.

25 QUESTIONS FOR SOCIAL SURVIVAL IN A PANDEMIC

In reality, the 25 questions and answers that follow are but a hint of the problems caused by pandemics and shelter-in-place on a social and educational scale. The list is limitless but here we begin it.

1. **If I am alone during the time that one must shelter-in-place, how do I not feel cut off from the world?**

   Today we have several options, all of which help but none of which are perfect solutions. Here are some ways to feel less alone:

   - Be creative in your use of technology. Interactive programs such as Zoom, Skype or FaceTime allow us to communicate without touching another person or being contagious.

- Listen to the radio, television, etc. Background noise helps to defeat the deafening silence of being alone or feeling cut off from the world.
- Go out for walks or drives. Even if you are not interacting with other people does not mean that you cannot see other people, and just seeing others, if from a distance, helps.

2. **What are some simple survival skills that I can use during a pandemic?**
   - Never lose your dignity. Even if you are alone establish a schedule and follow it. Dress as if others were seeing you and have regular mealtimes.
   - Make use of technology so that you do not feel disconnected from the world.
   - Take one or more on-line courses; learn something new.
   - Create lists of things that need to be done each day and do them.
   - Eat and sleep as if you were not in isolation.

3. **What are some things that I should avoid doing while in a shelter-in-place situation?**
   - Don't give up on personal hygiene. For example shower, shave, and pay attention to your body's details.
   - Don't become a hermit.
   - Don't turn down zoom or online invitations.

- Don't fail to share your feelings with those with whom you are living.
- Don't gossip.

4. **If I am at home with young children, how do I keep them from fighting?**
   This is an age-old question and family isolation tends to exacerbate difficult situations. Here are a few tips to consider:
   - Know when to hear and when not to hear.
   - Develop a plan to keep children occupied.
   - Develop plans for them to have alone time. Too much free time devolves quickly into turbulence.
   - Make each day a special day. Declare family holidays and have the children work together and separately on the "event of the day."

5. **How do I (we) as a parent(s) maintain order in the home?**
   Order starts with adult leadership. If adults are disorganized and slovenly then expect the same from children. Children learn from examples and an orderly home is a sign of dignity and mutual respect. As hard as it is, tidy up the home each day, insist that beds are made and that trash is taken out on time, and that dirty dishes are cleaned and put away.

6. **Are there psychological exercises that can help me get through the isolation?**

There is no secret formula. An article in the *Pursuit of Happiness* website titled "The Pursuit of Happiness and Positive Psychology" provides seven habits appropriate for these difficult times. They are:

- Deepen relationships with other people.
- Do something kind each day for others.
- Take care of yourself by eating well and exercising daily.
- Have goals and work toward them.
- Connect the spiritual and religion to your actions. Find a greater meaning to your life.
- Find your personal strengths and develop them to the utmost.
- Refuse to allow negative thoughts to destroy your life. Turn the negative into optimism, and gratitude.

7. **How much about a pandemic situation should I share with children?**

A great deal depends on your children and your relationship with them. Do not scare them nor exaggerate the situation. For most children the best is to explain the situation in clear and precise terms and reassure them that the government and you are doing everything possible to keep them safe and healthy. Dwell on positives, more family time, rather than negatives.

8. **How do I maintain educational levels without brick and mortar schools?**

Much of this answer depends on the educational levels of the children's parents and the parents' free time. Emphasize what you know rather than what you do not know. Make a plan and try to learn new things together as a family. For example, on the Internet study types of plants that are native to your part of the world and then go on a nature hunt.

Many families are now creating "educational pods." The families become "clans" where all members have been tested for the disease in question and then create "one room schoolhouses" where parents share their expertise with the children in the pod. The pod system allows for safe socialization experiences and a wider variety of learning opportunities.

9. **How much technology or computer time is too much?**
When the technology (be it a smart phone or the Internet) becomes addictive or becomes more important than human contact, then it is time to pull back.

10. **How do I substitute family activities for lack of friends?**
We do not have to give up our friends during a pandemic; we have only to give up the way we interacted in the past. Because of the wonders of technology, even during a full lockdown we can create "interactive play dates"

and adult friends can have virtual lunches or coffees together. During the COVID-19 crisis people took two meters-apart (six feet apart) walks, created on-line book clubs and discussion groups and new games based on the principles of social distancing.

11. **How important is a personal or family schedule?**

    Having a daily schedule is essential for a number of reasons. The following are among these:

    - A schedule maintains a sense of order in the home; don't do things in a helter-skelter fashion.
    - It allows everyone to have a sense of normalcy rather than be in a permanent state of crisis.
    - By reviewing the schedule each day each person can see what they accomplished or failed to finish and provides a sense of accomplishment and thereby an improved sense of being.

12. **Should I insist that everyone get "dressed" when staying at home?**

    Yes, staying in one's pajamas or sleeping clothes all day eventually leads to lethargy and a sense of ennui. It is best to maintain one's self-respect and one way to do this is by staying as close as possible to a regular schedule, not a "shelter-in-place" schedule. No matter what the circumstances might be, never lose your dignity.

13. **I feel frustrated and alone, can I choose to be happy or is that a matter of circumstance?**
    Happiness is a choice we make. Kathryn Sandford of *Lifehack* wrote this: "Is happiness a choice? Yes. But being happy requires more than just making the choice that 'I choose to be happy.' Sustaining happiness in your life takes commitment, courage, a deep understanding of that you are and knowing your purpose in life; and this does not happen overnight. It is a lifelong journey. By choosing to embrace happiness into your life, you are taking responsibility for your own contentment." *Goodreads* gives us these two quotes; first, Anne Frank wrote, "Our lives are fashioned by our choices. First we make our choices. Then our choices make us." And Albert Einstein summed it up best when he said that "There are two ways to live. You can live as if nothing is a miracle. You can live as if everything is a miracle."

14. **What are some things I can do to increase my happiness during the pandemic?**
    There is not one magic formula for happiness. Instead each person will need to discover his or her own road to happiness. Below is a potpourri of ideas and suggestions. Pick a few that make the most sense to you and best fit your personal situation:

- Do not think only about yourself. The number one way to feel happy is to do for others. Find a service project, give to charity or, in whatever way possible, know that you are working to make the world a better place.
- Be active. Get up each morning and plan one or two activities. These can be physical or mental. The best is a combination of both.
- Get out of the house. Even if it means taking a walk at 5:00 a.m. in the morning, a change of atmosphere does everyone a great deal of good.
- Eat well. Make sure that you have a balanced diet and eat at regular mealtimes.
- Spirituality and prayer help. Remember it takes just as much energy to be negative as positive, and prayer is a much better use of your energy or time than is worry. Bottom line: worry always makes things worse.
- Interact with everyone. Quick social interactions, done at a social distance, help to destroy feelings of isolation. The old saying "never met a stranger who wasn't a friend" is an important motto when we are home alone or feeling isolated. Arthur Brooks, from Harvard University, teaches a course on happiness and his book *The Art of Happiness* is a must read. One of Brooks' key themes is that we need to focus on what we have rather than on what we lack.

15. **How do I create a give-and-take attitude among my household members when we are stuck at home?**
    The classical Israeli kibbutz can serve as a model to create household peace and lower resentments. One of the most difficult situations for an isolated family is for some members to feel that most of the household work is falling on one person's shoulders while others are not doing their part. To avoid this problem make a list of everything that needs to be done from household chores to paying bills. Then hold a family meeting and divide up the chores, possibly on a weekly basis. Then, each week people can renegotiate, trade duties, or find new creative ways to handle family problems.

16. **How do I keep from blaming others for errors that I commit or just happen?**
    Transferring guilt is both human and destructive. Most people are good at blaming others and excellent at excusing their own failings. Start by assuming that whatever happens is your fault. It might not be but, by asking the question "What was my part in the problem?" we shift the focus away from the blame game and enter into the problem solving game.

    The more interaction that takes place the greater the tendency to become frustrated with and angry with our "living mates." Try to create personal time for each person and remember that in 99% of cases the one thing in life that you will get is over it!

17. **How do I deal with life-cycle events while in a shelter-in-place situation?**
In many cases you will not be able to be present. Try to create events on Zoom or other social media platforms, expect less and be grateful for what we have. For example, Peter Tarlow's mother died during the height of the COVID-19 pandemic. Funerals were "illegal" in New Jersey in April of 2020 and the cemeteries were closed. We created an on-line funeral and mourning period. Was it perfect? No, but we understood that we were doing the best that we could, and that had to be enough.

18. **How do I motivate myself to get out of bed when I am going nowhere?**
Getting out of bed is essential. It is the basis of maintaining one's dignity and a sense of personal value. If you do not value yourself then others will not value you. Remember the words of Rabbi Hillel from the Mishnaic period when he stated this: "If I am not for myself then who will be for me? If I am only for myself then what am I and if not now then when?"

Create a weekly list of things that must be done and then divide them each day. Make sure that you follow a rigorous schedule and look for new and innovative ways to make your day one of creativity and hope rather than of despair.

19. **How do I maintain my sense of dignity when I have so little to do?**
    Reframe the question to “what else can I do?” It is hard to have dignity when one is doing nothing, so use your time creatively. Learn something new, enhance a skill, find a way to earn money via the internet. Turn downtime into ‘uptime’ by doing something new each day such as learning a new language, or a new skill. The bottom line is stay busy and be creative.

20. **How do I control my anger?**
    Anger often comes from feeling out of control. So the number one way to control anger is to get over control issues. In reality none of us are really ever in control. All of us suffer disappointment and all of us probably believe that we are victims of something or someone. Victimization never leads to positive results but only to more anger. Take charge of what you can in your life and, as to the rest, simply realize that no one gets through life without problems. Focus on what you do have rather than what you lack.

21. **How do I keep from getting angry over trivial issues?**

Ask yourself: "Will this matter in two hours, two days or two months?" Most likely whatever happened that you chose to become angry over, will simply not matter. Most people often get angry when they turn the trivial into a major issue. Instead think about how trivial the issue is, learn to be stupid, and how to forget. You will be a lot happier.

22. **Is there a way that I can predict what will make me angry so as to avoid these issues before they occur?**
Get to know yourself. Being at home is a great time to keep notes. Each time you get angry write it down and then, after each week, patterns will begin to emerge. Once you have an idea as to what sets you off and makes you angry you can begin to deal with those issues and discover ways to avoid negative situations.

23. **How do we explain to children that right now money is tight and we will have to pull in our belts?**
Be honest. Children sense problems and not knowing is worse than being told the truth. Be frank but reassuring. Let children know that you all are together and that one way or another your family is going to be O.K. However, do not over promise, but be realistic and gentle at the same time.

24. **How do I find personal time when I am never alone?**
    Personal time should be included into family schedules. It might be only going for a short walk but personal time is almost as essential as eating. It is one of the best ways to control situations that seem out of control. Have a family meeting and schedule personal time, even of this time means nothing more than each person going to his or her room for twenty or thirty minutes a day.

25. **If we take a family road trip how do we maintain order while on the road?**
    If being in a house is difficult, being on a road trip requires lots of planning. If you are going to have to spend the night at a hotel or motel make sure that you check it out prior to arrival. What are their disease sanitation polices? What activities will there be for the children? Are there take out restaurants nearby? What will your rest room situation be? Then plan the trip, who will sit where? What toys, electronics and books will the parents need to entertain the children? How long will you drive between stops? Consider these three things on a road trip:
    - Games and toys
    - Quiet times
    - Food experiences

    If you are going by air then even greater planning might be needed. Air trips tend to be shorter but you don't have the flexibility of a car. That means that you are on the airline's schedule and assuming no delays. There's also the greater risk of contagion while traveling by air than by your own vehicle.

Delayed and cancelled flights can become a real challenge when traveling with children during the best of times. During a pandemic they can become even more of a challenge. Many people have decided therefore to turn a three-hour flight into a two-day road trip instead. Although a road trip is not easy it allows greater flexibility in what you can take with you and allows for more precise planning.

▪ ▪ ▪

Being together during a lockdown is not easy. Although lockdowns are hardest on the poor and the elderly, no one finds them to be enjoyable.

These are times that force us to be creative and innovative. Never ask too much of yourself and give yourself permission to feel the full range of emotions. Human beings are social animals, and we need each other.

Although social distancing, family lockdowns and separations are not easy, the bottom line is that we had no choice. Just as the British had to display a great deal of collective and personal fortitude during their darkest days of World War II, so too our generation has had to learn to creatively stand up to a different type of war.

Ours was a war where a virus viciously attacked millions of people around the world. Although we did not suffer bombs falling on our homes we too had to learn to deal with fear and uncertainty and discover our families and ourselves.

CHAPTER

5

PANDEMIC FINANCIAL STRESSES

ALTHOUGH A PHYSICIST would disagree with the statement that money moves the world—from a personal, political, and social perspective—money is an artificial force that plays fundamental importance in the development of humanity, heavily impacting human interactions and its relationships with the environment.

The economic crisis caused by the COVID-19 pandemic is another example of the interaction between wellness and wealth. During the pandemic millions of people lost their jobs and for some even their homes. Wealth, its accumulation and preservation became one of the topics of the day. Money concerns were so ubiquitous that the people-on-the-street talked more about money than even politics or sports. Ever since humans have understood the concept of wealth, and wanted to accumulate it and preserve it, there has been some form of seeking of wealth.

Wealth has come in many forms: the holding of land or animals, the possession of goods ranging from slaves to jewelry, the interchange of metallic commodities and then its replacement first by paper money and then by digitized symbols that represent money.

In our twenty-first century world the concept *money* as a form of exchange is ubiquitous. It is so ubiquitous that we take money's physical or digital existence almost for granted. No matter what the historical period might be, human beings have wanted to both grow and preserve their assets.

We might call this interaction with wealth "finances." Finances are what we do with our money regarding the way that we preserve it, grow it and utilize it. On a micro level, how we manage our finances can mean a life with less worry and more independence of action.

Unfortunately, popular society has transmitted several popular misconceptions about money. Often these misperceptions impact our personal and family lives. Humans created money to facilitate trade and commerce, that is to improve the quality of life. Instead of bartering goods, money allows freedom of access to essential and non-essential. Without some standard form of exchange, this access would be impossible. Money is an essential resource that must be watched over just as we would husband any other resource.

Money then can be both a source of "freedom" and a source of problems, or even psychological imprisonment. If not handled properly it can create distorted relationships leading to great personal vulnerability. Our lack of education in how to manage and handle money can lead to personal disaster and a life of eternal dissatisfaction.

Finances touch everyone's lives; they even touch small children's lives. For example any child who has ever received an allowance or opened up a lemonade stand is already involved in the business of finances.

On a macro level, how a large corporation handles its finances will determine not only its business model but also its success. On national and international levels, finances are a factor in tax rates, goods and services provided to a nation's citizens, and in the form of resource control. The handling of finances might mean the difference between war and peace.

FINANCIAL STRATEGIES FOR PANDEMIC TIMES

On a personal (micro) level, there are three things discussed below (call them strategies, actions, or habits) to assimilate into your life to fare better during a protracted crisis.

Learn to Take Calculated Risks

You will not get out of your situation if you carry on repeating the actions you have always been doing before.

In times of pandemics, it is clear that there are many variables that you are unable to control. This situation of high volatility, economic crisis, creates a perfect environment for you to step out of your "comfort" zone.

"Necessity is the mother of invention," Plato said. After the first shock of a job loss, of a massive decrease in revenue in your business, you have the opportunity to use your brain to innovate your life and maybe do what you never dared to do before.

Ensure that you take calculated risks, putting your financial safety first. The positive aspect of a crisis means that there is a reshuffle in how money flows. Look at this scenario as a new opportunity.

Learn to Invest in Yourself First

It is very difficult for you to create wealth in your life if you have not invested in yourself. Investing in yourself means dedicating time to yourself, to your learning, to your education, to your own development. Without that investment, your perception of personal worth is likely to be low, unless you were born into an extremely privileged position.

Building resilience is achieved by focusing on yourself and also by carefully selecting people around you who support you in your endeavors, learning and achievements.

Invest in yourself and your future, feed your mind with new teachings, and find honest mentors or coaches to support you as you turn things around.

Learn to Choose Education, Professional Help and Advice

When getting support, mentoring or advice be careful and extremely mindful so that ultimately you make decisions without being heavily influenced. Here are some pointers for specific situations:

- If you are an immigrant or someone who does not know much about your rights where you live, find someone competent who can help you with your situation.

- If you are thinking of starting a business and you are inexperienced in this, find a business mentor and surround yourself with a supportive network.

- When choosing a mentor, ensure that you share similar values. The relationship can work beautifully only as long as there are clear goals and a true willingness from your side to learn from the mentor you chose.

WHAT (GOOD) IS MONEY?

Before we ask questions about our own finances in a time of pandemic, let us take a moment to consider what money is and what it represents. If we strip away all of the things that people say about money, or all of the things that we have learned either formally or informally about money, we soon learn that money is nothing more than a symbolic form of energy.

Money is not good or bad; it simply is. The good or bad about money is not the money itself but how we choose to earn and invest it, how we chose to spend it, and how we handle it.

The University of Hawaii's College of Tropical Agriculture and Human Resources (CTAHR) notes this concept where it states that "Money means more than the coin, paper, or plastic to acquire goods and services. Money is linked to complex emotions, feelings, and behaviors. Each person has 'money messages' that are based on past experiences, what you observed and what you were taught. These money messages reflect the attitudes, perceptions, and expectations that influence your financial behaviors today."

Money represents the value of our "stored" energy as translated into a numerical term. Money symbolizes how we value our labor and the labor of others; it tells us what society in general and we in particular consider essential and what we do not. As we discuss our finances we are also discussing more than mere numbers but symbols of how we choose to live our lives and the values that we hold. During a time of pandemic, only our basic health takes on greater importance than the pursuit of money and our need to preserve it.

Although finances touch both the macro and the micro levels of society, this chapter focuses in on the personal and family level. Finances are often the source of personal anxiety and family frustrations, and once it is connected to a lack of morals and greed it can be a major motivator for crime. In fact, crime is a business that often destroys people's personal and family lives.

> "Money is not good or bad; it simply is. The good or bad about money is not the money itself gut how we choose to earn and invest it, how we choose to spend it, and how we we handle it.... [It] symbolizes how we value our labor and the labor of others ... [and what we] consider essential and what we do not."

The COVID-19 pandemic has increased many individuals' worries regarding their financial situation. After several months into the pandemic we know that people are not only suffering due to illnesses but also due to the impact of COVID-19 on national and personal economies. For example, the British Broadcasting Company (BBC) reported in June of 2020: "The International Monetary Fund has lowered its global growth forecast for this year [2020] and next in the wake of the coronavirus pandemic. It now predicts a decline of almost 5% in 2020, substantially worse than its forecast only 10 weeks ago in April."

Most people, however, are less worried about the international economy than they are about their own personal finances. Just as in politics, all finances are local.

As we noted in this book's introduction, the COVID-19 pandemic has impacted some people harder than others. Those who could work from home felt little financial strain due to the loss of a paycheck. On the other hand, families with young children had to combine work with childcare.

These people, however, were the lucky ones. Despite social strains caused by the pandemic, they were able to pay bills and avoid going into (additional) debt. On the other hand, there are millions of people who lost their jobs and incomes, and many independent businesses faced bankruptcy. Additionally, unfortunately, many of the people who lost their jobs (or were laid off) live from paycheck to paycheck. For those people, the situation is dire. They simply lack the savings and/or other streams of income to withstand a long financial setback or crisis.

Business and academic data bear out the extent of this problem. For example, in an article published in January of 2020 or a month prior to COVID-19 being on the horizon, MarketWatch noted that "Depending on the survey, that figure runs from half of workers making under $50,000 (according to Nielson data) to 74% of all employees (per recent reports from both the American Payroll Association and the National Endowment for Financial Education.) And almost three in 10 adults have no emergency savings at all, according to Bankrate's latest Financial Security Index. Even many in the upper class are seeing their six-figure incomes slip through their fingers. The Nielsen study found that one in four families making $150,000 a year or more are living paycheck-to-paycheck, while one in three earning between $50,000 and $100,000 also depend on their next check to keep their heads above water."

It should be emphasized that these figures reflect the financial situation prior to the onslaught of COVID-19 and the loss of jobs by millions of people.

Money Affects Our Perspectives

Our finances are windows into the practical side of the soul and reflect many of our views on life. No matter how much or how little money we might have, the way that we handle our money tells us much about who we are, and the values that we hold. From that perspective our finances are reflections of our values and core beliefs about life, and these are the essential values during a pandemic.

A crisis situation, such as a pandemic, tells us a

great deal about ourselves, and the ways we have chosen to live. Our financial management skills, or lack of skills, teach us a great deal about how we face risk, how we prepare for the future and if we seek immediate gratification. The way that we handle our money provides us with multiple insights into the way that we choose to organize our lives. It is not uncommon to discover that people whose finances are disorganized or in shambles also have disorganized or disoriented lives.

Learning to Put Personal Dignity Beyond Money

Personal worth can often be perceived as money, and affect our own perception of personal dignity. There are many reasons why you could be less well off or have financial struggles, that could also include your personal incapacity to manage finances, but not necessarily.

We are all born into different families and with different social backgrounds and opportunities. Some parents are able to teach their children important basics of law and finance, as well as promoting risk taking and entrepreneurial skills, while others do not.

Hence you might feel more or less privileged, more or less knowledgeable, more or less educated than others. Like or not humans have the natural tendency to compare themselves and, according to your social background, your gender, your ethnicity, the financial standing of your family at your moment of birth, you might have unnecessarily been treated in a more or less favorable way. In many cases these realities lead to a distorted personal perception of our self-worth, either inflated or deflated.

Whatever situation you recognize yourself to be in, building resilience is about seeing your dignity beyond what were or were not your privileges and financial achievements. Remember that—

- If you find yourself in financial difficulty and it is the result of the pandemic, you have the ability to build your success again.

- If you were in financial difficulty before and your finances were already disorganized, you now have the possibility to start afresh. Focus on developing yourself, your learning and your goals, as well as your personal well-being.

Building resilience means that you overcome the obstacles that you have in front of you. Like your body can learn to build defenses and antibodies to fight diseases, your mind can learn new ways of handling your finances. You can educate yourself and aim higher. Your ability to make money in the future depends also on your sense of personal worth, your dignity, and your perception of yourself.

▪ ▪ ▪

25 QUESTIONS ABOUT MONEY ISSUES IN A PANDEMIC

Many financial issues are not unique to a time of pandemic but they are always a concern; thus, these twenty-five questions refer to money and financial matters in general while some touch directly on financial resilience during a pandemic.

1. **How satisfied am I with the way I handle my money?**
   The answer to this question of course is personal. A good way to answer it is to also ask yourself: What do I need financially? Can I afford to satisfy my family's and my personal basic needs? If not, then you probably are not handling your money well. If you are borrowing money or dipping into savings on a regular basis, then you might want to adjust your spending to your earning capacities.

2. **If I were to lose my job due to a cause beyond my control such as a pandemic, how would I survive financially?**
   This question should be one of the first questions that you answer. What is the state of your savings? Do you have another profession to fall back on? Many of the questions that you will find below will help you answer this question and help to provide you with the knowledge needed to create a financial plan for both the good times and hard times.

3. **Do people younger than 40 need to save regularly?**
   Yes. It is unclear how long social security will last and what cuts might be made. Bottom line: never depend on a government agency to do for you what you should do for yourself.

4. **How solvent is social security*?**
   Of course no one can be sure, but prior to the COVID-19 pandemic U.S. government analysts predicted that social security would run dry by 2035. Of course this prediction is based on the current data and there might be changes such as higher taxes or money that is being spent on one item being transferred to another.

   The on-line journal *Investipedia* disagrees and notes that "Social Security is nowhere near bankruptcy. As Alicia H. Munnell, director of the Center for Retirement Research at Boston College, put it in her analysis of the 2017 annual report from the Board of Trustees: Social Security faces a manageable financing shortfall over the next 75 years, which should be addressed soon to share the burden more equitably across cohorts, restore confidence in the nation's major retirement program, and give people time to adjust to needed changes. If there is no fix in

* The term social security as used in this book refers to the U.S. government savings program that was developed during the 1930 Great Depression. It does not refer to any program outside the U.S.

the next 20 years, reduced benefits could be still paid with pay-as-you-go tax revenue. However, the sooner Congress does pass a fix and makes Social Security solvent, the better it will be for all of us." (Epstein). Without a healthy Social Security system the next health crisis will be that much worse.

5. **How much cash should I have on hand?**
   Prior to the COVID-19 pandemic it was believed that most people would do well to have at least three months of salary on hand. Today the rule of thumb is closer to six or nine months of saved income. A simple way to figure out how much money you will need is to add up all of your monthly expenses (not income) and then multiply the total number by three. Be sure to include easy-to-overlook costs like taxes, mortgage fees, car payments etc. Families with small children or senior citizens may want to change the three-month rule to six months.

6. **Has COVID-19 caused a unique financial crisis?**
   The answer here is yes and no. This crisis is different from the Great Depression of the 1930s in that it combines a health crisis with a financial crisis. Prior to January 2020 growth in the service industries and the travel and tourism industries offered many opportunities, espe-

cially for young people.

Suddenly all that changed. Over the following six months the U.S. economy contracted by almost a third, the travel and tourism industries were decimated, and many people in such professions as retail and service industries lost their jobs. It will take years to determine if these jobs are returning or if new jobs will have to be found.

Europe might have an even harder time as it is more reliant on regulations, has a disconnect between economic policy (set by the EU) and political policies (set by the home countries) and is less flexible in its ability to change quickly.

7. **Is it wise to invest in the stock market during a pandemic?**

Traditionally the stock market has outperformed other financial instruments, but there are several caveats that must be considered. Among these are the following:

- You can lose money in the stock market. Do not invest what you cannot afford to lose.
- The stock market might be down when you need the money. It is not a bank where money can be taken out or put in at will.
- The older you get the less time you will have to recover losses.
- Consider the advantages and disadvantages of mutual funds versus single stocks.

- Make sure that you have your basics covered before investing (gambling) in the stock market.
- Finally, the stock market could be in a "bear" (depressed)market during a pandemic, so act accordingly.

8. **If I am an older person (about to retire or retired) should I have money in the stock market?**

The information given above should help you make that decision. Older people face two threats: inflation that eats away at fixed incomes, and dips in the stock market when they need the money.

Ironically, the best way to handle these threats is with another threat. That is to say, that the stock market has been the best hedge against inflation, but it's also the least stable method to save money.

One way to deal with this problem is to determine what are one's essential expenses and place money for these essential needs into a less volatile savings plan, such as a bank. Use the stock market to save for luxury non-essential items such as a vacation.

On the other hand, during the last few years inflation has outpaced the interest paid by most banking institutions. This means that money in a bank account loses value during times of inflation.

9. **What do we mean by a balanced portfolio?**

   A balanced portfolio indicates that you have a mix of such instruments as stocks, bonds, real estate, commodities like gold or silver, and cash. Most people begin their portfolios by purchasing a house. But remember the house is not yours until you have paid off the mortgage. In the meantime you are building equity. The purchase of other forms of wealth will depend on your tolerance for risk and your financial responsibilities.

10. **How can I measure my resilience to financial risk?**

    There is no one method but we provide you with a "fun" quiz. Remember this is not scientific; it is merely a way to loosely gauge your readiness to survive financial stresses. That said, ask yourself the following questions and use the table below to score your answers:

    - Do you understand investing?
    - Is your job/source of income stable?
    - Do you own your home? (To own means to not owe money on a mortgage that could be foreclosed for non-payment)
    - In case of need do you feel comfortable that you will be able to access your assets should you have a personal financial crisis?
    - Do you have a business retirement plan?

- Are you free of extraordinary life expenses in the near future (such as caring for a parent or having another child)?
- Does your income meet your current needs without borrowing against credit cards?

ANSWERS	FINANCIAL RESILIENCE	COMMENT
0–1 Yes	Dangerously inadequate	In urgent need of correction
2–3 Yes	Inadequate	Reevaluate your strategies
4 Yes	Moderately adequate	Seek strategies to lower risk
5–6 Yes	Resilient	You are managing finances well
7 Yes	Exceptionally resilient	Among the lucky few

11. **How would a "bear market" impact the essential parts of my life, such as my housing, my children's education, or my ability to provide food and medicine for my family?**

    The way that you answer the questions above will help you determine your level of risk tolerance. Never put into an "investment" money that you cannot afford to lose. On the other hand, to do nothing is also a choice, and currently banks pay less interest than even the low rate of inflation. During the COVID-19 pandemic many people noticed that food prices increased by about 20%. This means that money in the bank lost about a fifth of its purchasing power.

12. **What is a mortgage?**
A mortgage is a loan made that allows you to purchase a home. Most mortgages are for 30 years of less. In the United States you pay the interest first and then build equity, thus additional payments at the beginning of a mortgage saves the borrower a great deal of money and cuts years off the life of the loan.

13. **Is it wise to own real estate?**
Most people own at least some real estate if they have purchased a home. But purchasing a home does not mean owning a home. As long as you have a mortgage the mortgage lender owns your home. Additionally, each year you must pay property taxes and failing to do so could result in the loss of a home.

Real estate has often been seen as a good balance to stocks and bonds. It is a tangible asset. To make money, however, you have to rent the real estate to another person and should there be a lack of renters then you will be paying taxes and upkeep with no additional income. During the COVID-19 pandemic the U.S. government said that people could not be evicted for lack of rental payment. In cases where home renters could not pay the rent the landlord has to assume expenses, such as taxes, without compensation.

14. **How much debt can I tolerate?**
Families are not nations and cannot print money. That means that if the cost of servicing the debt (and that includes fixed debts such as rent, mortgage and car payments) and covering expenses is greater than income, the family has a major problem and bankruptcy will occur. During the COVID-19 crisis many families could not afford their car payments and these defaults meant that there was a glut of pre-owned vehicles.

15. **Do I need a financial advisor?**
The more complicated your finances the more you need an advisor. Most people have not studied (or do not remember) the basic principles of finance. It is a lot cheaper to pay a specialist than it is to make financial mistakes. Make sure that you find a competent and honest advisor and then listen to their advice. One of the tasks of a good financial advisor will be to help you understand your finances, your liabilities, your short term and long term needs, and to establish realistic financial goals. If you are careful about your medical advisor the same holds true for a financial advisor. Do not be afraid to ask questions and get a second opinion.

16. **How often should I review my financial goals?**
    Most financial advisors want to have at least a yearly review of your finances. As you get closer to retirement age, and once in retirement age, you should meet at least twice a year. During periods of financial instability such as a pandemic you might need to meet on a quarterly basis with telephone meetings as needed. Just as in the case of medicine, as you get older your should increase the number of times that you review your financial health.

17. **During a pandemic what lessons should I teach my children about money?**
    Perhaps the most important lesson is that nothing in life is guaranteed. During times of prosperity prepare for difficult times. Families with financial reserves do a lot better than those without. Therefore starting as children we need to learn the importance of money, how to handle it and how to preserve it.

18. **During the pandemic and at no fault of their own, my teenagers have lost their outside job. How do I continue to teach them the value of work?**
    This is a great example of turning lemons into lemonade. Chat with them about the importance of flexibility, of savings and of having a skill. They are learning that life is not always

fair and that they need to have the skill sets and education to be able to survive in this world. Use the layoff as an opportunity to do a skills inventory and also for them to think about how they want to shape their future.

19. **Should a pandemic force us to develop a family budget?**
    Yes! During a pandemic, especially if the pandemic has caused one or more members of a family to lose a job, everyone has to pitch in. Use the pandemic as a way to learn to work together and find ways to allow everyone to chip in, be that by cutting expenses or by increasing income. Being part of a family budget not only makes children feel part of a family but also acts as an empowerment tool. Instead of being merely a leaf floating through the air with no direction, the family budget allows people a sense that they have control over their own lives.

20. **How do I determine which financial data are correct and which are not?**
    There is a great deal of information out there. Don't accept any one source, especially from the Internet. Not everything on the Internet is true. First, speak to a trusted and certified financial advisor, then read multiple sources and distinguish between rumors and facts. Sources such as Forbes and the Wall Street

Journal often provide hard facts. No matter what, never allow anyone to pressure you into something that does not feel right.

21. **Will the 2020 pandemic lead to a depression or long-term economic scenario?**
Of course, no one knows for certain the correct answer to this question. Part of the answer depends on how long and severe the pandemic lasts, which party's financial plans are put in place, and if therapeutic methods or vaccines are discovered to bring the virus to its end. These are unknowns.

The other unknown is if a pandemic is part of a biological attack, or something that occurred without malice of forethought. Currently both the United States and the European Union are taking extraordinary measures to prevent a financial collapse, but they are also printing a great deal of money that might lead to a period of major inflation.

22. **How is the stock market different now than during the Great Depression?**
Hindsight is always seen with 20/20 vision. We know what we did wrong during the Great Depression and we think we know how to prevent repeating that history. The 1929 crash started a massive deflation because the Federal Reserve did not cut interest rates sufficiently and that caused the stock market to lose 86%

of its worth when inflation soared to 16%.

Today we are seeing the exact opposite occurring and we have to hope that the mistakes of the past have been factored into the current crisis. By the end of 2021 around $5 trillion dollars will have been added to the economy and the Central Banks in Europe, the U.K. and Japan have followed some form of quantitative easing. It's hoped that these policies will prevent a repeat of the 1930s.

23. **How do I pay my taxes if I am out of a job?**

In the United States the Internal Revenue Service (IRS) has shown a certain amount of understanding. However, governments want money and compassion only goes so far. It might be wise to speak with an accountant, understand what your tax burden will be and then budget your tax burden into your family budget. That way, should you have to pay additional taxes you will have the necessary funds.

24. **How do I handle child support when I am out of work?**

Most civil courts consider child support your first priority. Their argument is that a child comes first. This argument comes at a cost, especially if the person paying child support has to maintain a second family or if the person receiving the child support uses the money for some other reason. It is a good idea to consult a family practice lawyer and then go to the courts as soon as possible and learn what options exist and what can be done during these difficult days.

25. **Given all of the uncertainty and all that I have learned in this chapter, should I be afraid?**

    In the end, fear solves nothing. Instead review all of your assets and create a balance between real estate, stocks and bonds, commodities etc. Then develop a family budget in which you do not spend more than you have and find ways to cut expenses by ten percent. If you can reduce debt (or eliminate it) and have balanced your assets you should be fine, and you might even find some wonderful financial opportunities.

    The bottom line is that we all need to base our financial decisions on facts and not on emotions. Obtain the best advice available and do not spend what you do not have. If you use a commonsense approach to finance you should weather the storm well.

■ ■ ■

Perhaps there are few aspects of our lives that create as much stress as finances. Financial stress plays a role in many people's lives be they rich or poor. As we have seen in this chapter, the best ways to avoid stress are to save and invest during the good times and plan for the hard times. Never purchase what you cannot afford, learn to live within a budget, and realize that the world of finances is a complicated world. Do not be afraid to ask questions and to learn.

Money may not move the world but if we are not careful with our finances then it will certainly make our heads spin!

CHAPTER

6

EPILOGUE

THIS BOOK IS more than merely about personal resilience due to the Covid-19 crisis. It is about personal resilience no matter what the crisis might be. The Covid-19 pandemic might have been the first worldwide health crisis since the misnamed Spanish flu of 1918, but with modern transportation and an ever-more globalized world, the odds are that it might well not be the last. It's for this reason that we need to develop the *social antibodies of personal resilience.* Just as the body cannot recover from an illness without antibodies, so too we each must find the strength of character needed to survive the crisis and to go beyond its confines.

We define personal resilience as the result of the constant process of not giving up—and transforming a world challenge into an opportunity for personal growth. It is the perennial challenge of turning lemons into lemonade, and danger into opportunity.

Illnesses such as Covid-19 require a fighting spirit. We know that diseases are not stable; they can evolve, modify, or disappear, or attack us, or decide to leave our bodies and our society in peace.

But what does it mean to have a fighting spirit? Different cultures offer insights into this question. For example, in Nichiren Buddhism, a fighting spirit is the ability to transform oneself and aspire to a higher state of being. Nichiren Buddhism sees every challenge as an opportunity to grow and develop into a better, stronger and more resilient being, a person who uses the crisis to become happier and more tranquil.

> " The COVID-19 pandemic … might well not be the last. It's for this reason that we need to develop *the social antibodies of personal resilience.*"

Christians might look to their Bible and quote from Corinthians 4:16-18. From their perspective the "eternal" weight of today might well become the opportunity of tomorrow. It is from this belief that a Christian might see the Covid-19 crisis as an opportunity for renewal.

Unfortunately, history has made Jews specialists in finding the strength to get through periods of pain and suffering. During the Holocaust, the apex of humanity's tragic failing, Viktor Frankl wrote that "When we are no longer able to change a situation, we are challenged to change ourselves."

If we are able to foster a fighting spirit and become more resilient we then have the possibility in the process to become a better version of ourselves: stronger, more determined, more decisive, and more focused on what you want.

Throughout this book we discussed how a pandemic affects different people in different ways. Inevitably lives are lost and grief is the feeling that we are left with.

In a sense, after Covid-19 is making us all survivors. As survivors, we can learn a huge amount about ourselves by living through these difficult times. How often do we appreciate what we had only after it's gone? The current pandemic has reduced our physical mobility: We no longer commute to work. During the pandemic travel seemed to become a "thing of the past."

Not all has been negative, though. For some the pandemic has provided additional family time, and the lack of travel has greatly improved the world's air quality. The need to stay home has allowed the planet to heal. In one example a few months ago, the picture of dolphins in the canals in Venice (Italy) were a sight which was heart-warming after the virus caused so many deaths there.

The pandemic has also shown many of us a different way of living: working from home is possible and efficient in some cases, and remote, online working and schooling still has many unexplored avenues for the future.

Building personal resilience means understanding the challenges of today and transforming them into the advantage of tomorrow.

Being faced by death and grief and by the inevitability of events that are completely out of our hands also gives us food for thought—they remind us that each day is a gift and to waste a moment of time is perhaps one of the great sins.

All events pass, but during this event take the time to ask yourself some new questions. If, at the time, you would have known what you know now—

Would you have done anything differently? If yes, what?

Could you have prepared yourself better?

What can you take from this analysis?

Self-analysis is a process which when done continuously and in a proficient way is especially useful. It is not about blaming yourself for your shortcomings, but more about realizing that at the time you did not know any better. We all make decisions based on the data that we have at that moment.

Resilience is the act of learning from mistakes and applying this knowledge to create a better future. We are all subject to situations that are beyond our control, such as the pandemic, a boss, a government or a higher authority. To be human is to recognize that we all have shortcomings and none of us is entirely in control. We might not have control over the events in our lives but we do control our reactions to these events.

In unprecedented situations such as a pandemic we all make mistakes. To be resilient is to turn these mistakes into wisdom and create opportunities from past life lessons.

Would you have really done something differently?

Are you aware of the limitations that were present at the moment? If so, could you do something about it?

We all have choices in life. How we choose to react is up to us. The apparently small changes we make today may be the ones that lead to a better future.

At almost the end of the book of Deuteronomy, just as the Children of Israel are about to enter into the land of Israel, Moses challenges each one of them with the following words:

> Behold I have set before each of you the choice of a blessing or a curse, choose life so that you and your offspring might live!"

To be resilient is to accept Moses' challenge and to choose life. It's for each of us to take ownership of the choices we make and plan for our future. It is incumbent upon each of us to protect ourselves from what we cannot control, learn from our previous mistakes and take the actions so that in the words of Moses you too shall have chosen life.

Works Cited

Al-Khateeb, Zac. "College Football Cancellations, Explained: Answering Questions on COVID-19 and What's Next for 2020 Season." *U.S. Sporting News*, 16 Aug. 2020, www.sportingnews.com/us/ncaa-football/news/college-football-canceled-2020-season-covid-19/1idsr90t6at3210k84n0x3rpds.

All About History. "Spanish Flu: The Deadliest Pandemic in History." *LiveScience*, Future US, Inc., 12 Mar. 2020, www.livescience.com/spanish-flu.html.

Begley, Sharon. "Desperate for Covid-19 Answers, U.S. doctors Turn to Colleagues in China." *STAT Magazine*, 24 Mar. 2020, www.statnews.com/2020/03/24/covid-19-answers-doctors-turn-to-china.

Bettinger-Lopez, Caroline. "A Double Pandemic: Domestic Violence in the Age of COVID-19." *Council on Foreign Relations*, 13 May 2020, www.cfr.org/in-brief/double-pandemic-domestic-violence-age-covid-19.

Braucher, David. "How to Survive 'Social Distancing' and 'Shelter in Place'." *Psychology Today*, 22 Mar. 2020, www.psychologytoday.com/us/blog/life-smarts/202003/

how-survive-social-distancing-and-shelter-in-place.

Breen, Kerry. "Can You Reuse a Disposable Mask? Yes, If You Follow These Steps." *Yahoo! News*, 14 Jul. 2020, www.news.yahoo.com/reuse-disposable-mask-yes-steps-192223361.html?guce_referrer_us=aHR0cHM6Ly93d3cuZ29vZ2xlLmNvbS8&guce_referrer_cs=CoinlsTiHj3J-MPo186EWg.

Brown, Dan and Elisabetta De Cao. "Child Maltreatment, Unemployment, and Safety Nets." *SSRN*, 19 Mar. 2020, www.papers.ssrn.com/sol3/papers.cfm?abstract_id=3543987.

CDC. "Coping With Stress." *Centers for Disease Control and Prevention*, U.S. Department of Health & Human Services, 22 Jan. 2021, www.cdc.gov/coronavirus/2019-ncov/daily-life-coping/managing-stress-anxiety.html.

—. "Food and Coronavirus Disease 2019." *Centers for Disease Control and Prevention*, U.S. Department of Health & Human Services, 31 Dec. 2020, www.cdc.gov/coronavirus/2019-ncov/daily-life-coping/food-and-COVID-19.html.

—. "Framework for Healthcare Systems Providing Non-COVID-19 Clinical Care During the COVID-19 Pandemic." *Centers for Disease Control and Prevention*, U.S. Department of Health & Human Services, 30 Jun. 2020, www.cdc.gov/coronavirus/2019-ncov/hcp/framework-non-COVID-care.html.

—. "How to Wear Masks." *Centers for Disease Control and Prevention*, U.S. Department of Health & Human Services, 30 Jan. 2021, www.cdc.gov/coronavirus/2019-ncov/prevent-getting-sick/how-to-wear-cloth-face-coverings.html.

Cohen, Elliot. "Your Are a Social Animal." *Psychology Today*, 21 Sep. 2010, www.psychologytoday.com/us/blog/what-would-aristotle-do/201009/you-are-social-animal.

De Cao, Elisabetta and Malte Sandner. "The Potential Impact of the COVID-19 on Child Abuse and Neglect: The Role of Childcare and Unemployment." *VOX EU*, Centre for Economic Policy Research, 8 May 2020, www.voxeu.org/article/potential-impact-covid-19-child-abuse-and-neglect.

Delagran, Louise. "What Is Spirituality?" *University of Minnesota*, Earl E. Bakken Center for Spirituality & Healing, www.takingcharge.csh.umn.edu/what-spirituality. Accessed 13 Mar. 2021.

Einstein, Albert. "Quotable Quote." *Goodreads*, Goodreads, Inc., "Quotable Quote." *Goodreads*, Goodreads, Inc., www.goodreads.com/quotes/987-there-are-only-two-ways-to-live-your-life-one. Accessed 22 Sep. 2020.

Epstein, Lita. "How Secure Is Social Security?" *Investopedia*, 26 Nov. 2020, www.investopedia.com/articles/personal-finance/120415/how-secure-social-security.asp.

Foley, Logan. "Sleep Guidelines During the COVID-19 Pandemic." *Sleep Foundation*, 17 Dec. 2020, www.sleepfoundation.org/sleep-guidelines-covid-19-isolation.

Frank, Anne. "Quotable Quote." *Goodreads*, Goodreads, Inc., www.goodreads.com/quotes/751625-our-lives-are-fashioned-by-our-choices-first-we-make. Accessed 22 Sep. 2020.

Huffman, Kevin. "Homeschooling During the Coronavirus Will Set Back a Generation of Children." *The Washington Post*, 27 Mar. 2020, www.washingtonpost.com/outlook/coronavirus-homeschooling-will-hurt-students-badly/2020/03/27/f639882a-6f62-11ea-b148-e4ce3fbd85b5_story.html.

Intermountain Healthcare. "What's the Difference Between a Pandemic, an Epidemic, Endemic, and an Outbreak?" *Intermountain Healthcare*, Live

Well, 2 Apr. 2020, www.intermountainhealthcare.org/blogs/topics/live-well/2020/04/whats-the-difference-between-a-pandemic-an-epidemic-endemic-and-an-outbreak.

King, Barbara. "Seeing Spirituality in Chimpanzees." *The Atlantic*, 29 Mar. 2016, www.theatlantic.com/science/archive/2016/03/chimpanzee-spirituality/475731.

Levere, Jane. "Airlines Say It's Safe to Travel. But Is It? *The New York Times*, 8 Jul. 2020, www.nytimes.com/2020/06/01/business/coronavirus-airports-airlines.html.

Lewin, Daniel. "COVID-19 and Healthy Sleep Habits." *Rise and Shine Magazine*, Children's National, 16 Apr. 2020, www.riseandshine.childrensnational.org/covid-19-and-healthy-sleep-habits.

Lindo, Jason M., et al. "Caution! Men Not at Work: Gender-Specific Labor Market Conditions and Child Maltreatment." *Journal of Public Economics*, vol. 163, 2018, pp. 77–98. *Crossref*, doi:10.1016/j.jpubeco.2018.04.007.

Liu, Yi-Ling. "Is Covid-19 Changing Our Relationships?" *BBC Future*, 4 Jun. 2020, www.bbc.com/future/article/20200601-how-is-covid-19-is-affecting-relationships.

Mahan, William. "How to Define Ethical Behavior & Why It's Important in the Workplace." *Work Institute*, 17 Oct. 2019, www.workinstitute.com/how-to-define-ethical-behavior-why-its-important-in-the-workplace-2.

Medalie, Lisa. "Why It's Important to Get a Good Night's Sleep During the Coronavirus Outbreak." *UChicago Medicine*, 16 Apr. 2020, www.uchicagomedicine.org/forefront/coronavirus-disease-covid-19/advice-for-sleeping-well-during-the-covid-19-outbreak.

My Accounting Course. "What Is Ethical Behavior?" *My Accounting Course*, MyAccountingCourse.com, www.myaccountingcourse.com/accounting-dictionary/ethical-behavior. Accessed 12 Dec. 2020.

"Noahide Laws." *New World Encyclopedia*, www.newworldencyclopedia.org/entry/Noahide_Laws. Accessed 21 Nov. 2020.

Owens, Amber L. "Through for Good." *familyfriend Poems*, FFP Inc., Feb. 2006, www.familyfriendpoems.com/poem/dad-and-mom-stop-fighting-through-for-good.

Puchalski, Christina. "The Role of Spirituality in Health Care." *U.S. National Library of Medicine*, National Center for Biotechnology Information, Oct. 2001 14(4): 352-357. DOI:10.1080/08998280.2001.1192788. www.ncbi.nlm.nih.gov/pmc/articles/PMC1305900.

Pursuit of Happiness. "The Science of Happiness and Positive Psychology." *Pursuit of Happiness,* Pursuit-of-Happiness.org. www.pursuit-of-happiness.org/science-of-happiness/?gclid=Cj0KCQjw6575BRCQARIsAMpksPdTD-ig9UvTxlYMtK5fwLQcoyklBty0FgAkIKTNeRL6Hvka4A1aHEaAsdsEALw_wcB. Accessed 23 Aug. 2020.

Sandford, Kathryn. "How to Always Choose Happiness Even During Tough Times." *Lifehack*, www.lifehack.org/828297/choose-happiness. Accessed 20 Feb. 2021.

Schaerfer, Dovovan. *Religious Affects: Animality, Evolution and Power.* Duke University Press, 2015.

"Spirituality." *Merriam-Webster.com Dictionary*, Merriam-Webster, www.merriam-webster.com/dictionary/spirituality. Accessed 21 Jun. 2020.

States Attorney. "Divorce Rates and COVID-19." *States Attorney,* StatesAttorney.org, 2 May 2020, www.statesattorney.org/2020/05/02/divorce-rates-and-covid-19.

Suni, Eric. "Sleep Guidelines During the COVID-19 Pandemic." *Sleep Foundation*, OneCare Media Company, 17 Dec. 2020, www.sleepfoundation.org/sleep-guidelines-covid-19-isolation.

Tarlow, Peter, et al. *Personal Reconstruction: A Psychological, Spiritual, Financial and Legal Course in the Art of Preventing Personal Crises, and Recovering From Them*. Quest Publishing, 2018.

Uliano, Sophie. "Self Awareness." *Pinterest*, www.pinterest.ca/pin/362047257528470566. Accessed 15 Mar. 2021.

UN Department of Economic and Social Affairs. "Everyone Included: Social Impact of COVID-19." *United Nations*, www.un.org/development/desa/dspd/everyone-included-covid-19.html. Accessed 27 Jun. 2020.

——. "Special Issue on COVID-19 and Youth." *United Nations*, 27 Mar. 2020, PDF from www.un.org/development/desa/dspd/wp-content/uploads/sites/22/2020/04/YOUTH-FLASH-Special-issue-on-COVID-19-1.pdf downloaded 27 Mar. 2021.

Van Kyk, Tori. "Healthy Sleep During COVID-19." *Loma Linda University School of Behavioral Health.*, May 12, 2020, www.behavioralhealth.llu.edu/blog/healthy-sleep-during-covid-19.

University of Minnesota. "What is Spirituality?" *University of Minnesota*, www.takingcharge.csh.umn.edu/what-spirituality. Accessed 21 Jun. 2020.

Walsch, Neale Donald. *Conversations with God: An Uncommon Dialogue, Book 1*. 1st ed., New York, G. P. Putnam's Sons, 1996.

Woodall, Candy. "As Hospitals See More Severe Child Abuse Injuries During Coronavirus, 'The Worst Is Yet To Come.'" *USA Today*, 13 May 2020, www.usatoday.com/story/news/nation/2020/05/13/hospitals-seeing-more-severe-child-abuse-injuries-during-coronavirus/3116395001.

About the Authors

Peter Tarlow, Ph.D.

Dr. Peter E. Tarlow is a world-renowned speaker and expert specializing in the impact of crime and terrorism on the tourism industry, event and tourism risk management, and tourism and economic development. He was also the director and rabbi of Texas A&M Hillel for thirty years. Upon retirement, he assumed the leadership of the Center for Latino – Jewish Relations.

Peter writes a weekly bilingual social religious commentary that is read throughout the United States and Latin America and he also writes a monthly philosophy column for the Bryan Eagle.

He has been a chaplain for the College Station police department since 1988, and in April of 2013, he was asked to accept the role of Envoy for the Office of Chancellor of the Texas A&M System, John Sharp. In 2015 he began teaching at the Texas A&M Medical School's Department of Humanities, and in 2016, Governor Gregg Abbot of Texas named him as the Chairman of the Texas Holocaust and Genocide Commission.

Séverine Obertelli

Séverine is an internationally respected speaker and expert who lectures on personal resilience and development. Her course touches on how we can promote physical, emotional, financial, and spiritual well-being practices. As a personal and business coach, she aids people from all walks of life to balance their careers, businesses, and family commitments. Séverine's teaching provides strategies for developing life balance and personal fulfillment. Her work has become especially important during these times of pandemics and lockdowns. Séverine teaches us how to use our values, spirituality, and faith to not only survive during a pandemic but to thrive.

Beyond her work with individuals, Séverine has worked with a wide range of international boards in the fields of tourism and hospitality. She emphasizes the need for collaboration and innovative thinking as tools to create greater social impact and accountability.

In the world of consulting Séverine is well-known for her innovation and organizational strategies and for helping entrepreneurs, business leaders, and corporate organizations to develop global impacts while enhancing their personal, social, and economic assets.

Acknowledgments

This book's authors want to acknowledge all whom the pandemics of 2020-2021 have impacted. We have written this book to help all who have suffered during this terrible pandemic. The book is for those whom the disease attacked, those who survived it, those whose families have lost loved ones, and those who have worked tirelessly to help others.

The COVID-19 pandemic touched both rich and poor, young and elderly, wise and simple. It serves as a reminder that humanity is one family living together on a small planet floating through the vastness of the universe. In that sense, the COVID-19 pandemic serves as a model for future medical challenges. On some level, it has taught us all that we are part of one human family.

We also realize that we would not have been able to succeed in this endeavor without the loving support of our families and their willingness to "sacrifice time" with us so we could accomplish this goal. Finally, we wish to acknowledge Jacques Island and his Quest Publishing colleagues without whose support this project would never have come to fruition.

Index

R

S

Lightning Source UK Ltd.
Milton Keynes UK
UKHW020704270621
386232UK00003B/14

9 780976 941644